Sensory Modulation in Dementia Care

of related interest

Adaptive Interaction and Dementia
How to Communicate without Speech
Dr Maggie Ellis and Professor Arlene Astell
Illustrations by Suzanne Scott
ISBN 978 1 78592 197 1
eISBN 978 1 78450 471 7

Visiting the Memory Café and other Dementia Care Activities
Evidence-based Interventions for Care Homes
Edited by Caroline Baker and Jason Corrigan–Charlesworth
Foreword by Dr G. Allen Power
ISBN 978 1 78592 252 7
eISBN 978 1 78450 535 6

Embracing Touch in Dementia Care
A Person-centred Approach to Touch and Relationships
Luke Tanner
ISBN 978 1 78592 109 4
eISBN 978 1 78450 373 4

Sensory Modulation in Dementia Care

Assessment and Activities for Sensory-Enriched Care

Tina Champagne

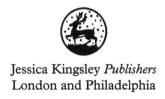

Jessica Kingsley *Publishers*
London and Philadelphia

First published in 2018
by Jessica Kingsley Publishers
73 Collier Street
London N1 9BE, UK
and
400 Market Street, Suite 400
Philadelphia, PA 19106, USA

www.jkp.com

Library of Congress Cataloging in Publication Data
A CIP catalog record for this book is available from the Library of Congress

British Library Cataloguing in Publication Data
A CIP catalogue record for this book is available from the British Library

ISBN 978 1 78592 733 1
eISBN 978 1 78450 427 4

Printed and bound by CPI Group (UK) Ltd, Croydon, CR0 4YY

In honor of my grandmother, who had dementia in the later years of her life. Her experiences inspired me to adapt the Sensory Modulation Program more specifically to working with people with dementia. She enjoyed many of the strategies proposed in this book. She also instilled in me the importance of helping others and of having a sense of humor, and always encouraged me to go after my dreams.

Contents

Conclusion 141

Acknowledgments

To my children, I am deeply grateful to you for your love and ongoing support. To Kristina Tams, thank you for helping with the editing of this book. To my mentors and colleagues, thank you for supporting my ideas and projects over the years; it has been wonderful to collaborate with all of you about how important it is to address sensory integration and processing, as part of occupational therapy and other therapeutic services, with different populations and in various settings. To those of you who have worked with me with this specific population (people with dementia), it has been an honor to work together to develop and implement approaches that have helped to demonstrate the value of a more humane, nurturing, compassionate, and sensory-based approach—thank you!

Thank you also to Karen Poole, TFH USA (www.tfhusa.com) and Lisa Compton (www.SensoryCraver.com) for granting permission to use the product photographs in this book.

About the Author

Tina Champagne, OTD, OTR/L, FAOTA, is the Executive Director of Cutchins Programs for Children and Families in Northampton, Massachusetts. She is also the director of and primary consultant for Champagne Conferences and Consultation, and a professor for the American International College's doctoral program in occupational therapy.

Dr. Champagne is an occupational therapist and her primary areas of interest include: organizational change, trauma and attachment informed care, the applicability of individualized, sensory-based approaches across the lifespan, mental health, wellness, and quality of life. She has published a variety of books, book chapters, articles, resource documents, and research studies.

Dr. Champagne is also a reviewer for several peer-reviewed journals and the creator of the Sensory Modulation Program. Dr. Champagne has received numerous awards and is highly recognized for her work, particularly in its application across a broad variety of practice settings and age ranges.

Introduction

Given the significant advancements in the field of neuroscience, it is now widely recognized that the different sensory-rich experiences human beings encounter every day help to "nourish the nervous system" (Ayres 1979, 2005). Each of the sensory systems has specialized receptors that detect very specific types of sensory stimuli. The sensory input received by the receptors is sent to the brain, and helps to support the ability to feel safe and self-regulated, and to functionally engage in meaningful roles, routines, and activities. The eyes detect and track visual and spatial input, the ears pick up on sounds, the nose takes in the air we breathe and different types of chemicals known to us as scents, and the skin contains a variety of tactile receptors that help us understand the many different types of touch sensation experienced (e.g., light touch pressure, deep touch pressure, temperature, vibration, pain). The mouth is used to taste, eat, and drink, and also to breathe, speak, sing, and even play an instrument!

In addition to the five basic sensory systems (tactile, vision, auditory, olfaction [smell], and gustatory [taste]), there are a few others that people rarely know about. These sensory systems are the vestibular, proprioceptive, and interoceptive systems. The vestibular system supports the ability to overcome gravity, coordinate the body, and safely navigate the world. Muscles are also major sensory organs and the proprioceptive receptors are located in the muscles, joints, tendons, and connective tissues of the body. The proprioceptive receptors are activated when a person engages in activities against resistance, stretching, or other movement-based actions. Proprioceptive input contributes to the ability to know where the body is in space and time from a body-based "felt" sense. The vestibular and proprio-ceptive systems work together with other sensory systems to support body awareness, equilibrium, and the ability to sequence the body through the different steps of activities. Interoception is the ability to be aware of one's different internal states (e.g., degrees of alertness, illness, hunger, digestion).

The processing and organization of all sensory and motor input is part of the role of the central nervous system across the lifespan. The way an individual processes and organizes sensory input contributes to the formation of one's self-perception, the perception of others, and the phys-ical environment. Different types and intensities of sensory and motor stimuli influence whether or not a person feels safe, regulated, and able to functionally communicate and engage in activities. In fact, without enough sensory input throughout each day sensory deprivation occurs, making it difficult for human beings to remain resilient and able to gain or maintain skills, such as strength, agility, and the ability to pay attention. The sensory systems also play a protective role, by sending signals to the brain that help to alert individuals to potential safety concerns.

Using a sensory-based approach with people with dementia requires focusing intentionally and strategically on the amounts and types of sen-sory stimuli a person experiences, in order to help maintain skills, support participation, and ensure safety, comfort, and quality of life. Exploring each person's sensory preferences and patterns, and identifying sensory-based needs and goals, is also part of a sensory-based approach. At times, sensory strategies are also used to help distract from pain, discomfort, and difficult thoughts (paranoia, confusion, ruminations) and emotions (anger, sadness, fear). Other times, sensory strategies may be used to help people feel calm, soothed, and comforted, and to promote feelings of safety and security. Sensory strategies may be used for compensatory purposes or to promote leisure and social participation. In addition, sensory strategies can be used to help decrease the incidence of agitation, aggressive behaviors, and the use of restraints.

In summary, this book provides a general overview of the different types of dementia, and an introduction to sensory integration and pro-cessing, the sensory systems, and how the functioning of the sensory systems may change as people age. Additionally, the Sensory Modulation Program (SMP) is presented as a comprehensive, non-pharmacological framework that may be used when caring for or working with people with dementia. The SMP is the most helpful when wanting to implement the use of a sensory-based approach in a comprehensive manner. For the purposes of this publication, the SMP has been adapted specifically for use with people with dementia.

Chapter 1

Aging and Dementia

The purpose of life is to live it, to taste experience to the utmost, to reach out eagerly and without fear for newer and richer experience.
~ Eleanor Roosevelt

Aging is a natural phenomenon among human beings. Although some people believe that dementia is a typical part of aging, the Alzheimer's Association (AA 2017a) reports that this belief is a myth. Many older adults are able to age without the onset of dementia. For those who do develop dementia, there are several different reasons why it may occur. This chapter reviews some of the general types of dementia, examples of reasons for its onset, and common safety considerations to keep in mind when caring for or working with someone with dementia. The information presented in this chapter is not all-inclusive and is meant to serve as an introduction to the topics covered.

According to the Alzheimer's Association (*ibid.*), dementia encompasses a variety of symptoms associated with a decline in memory, or other cognitive and thinking skills, which are severe enough to impact negatively the ability to remember friends and loved ones, and safely and functionally perform daily routines and activities. When someone has dementia, the disease and corresponding symptoms are *progressive*, which means the condition and related symptoms worsen over time. Depending upon the areas of the brain that are impacted, a variety of different kinds of cognitive, social, emotional, and functional challenges may emerge. Some of the common challenges for those with dementia occur across the following areas:

- Safety (e.g., fall risk, agitation/aggression, medical complications, physical injuries, wandering and getting lost)

- Cognition (e.g., memory, attention span, problem solving)

- Sensory acuity (e.g., changes in vision, hearing, taste)

- Sensory and motor integration and processing (e.g., deconditioning, balance problems, problems with spatial orientation, and decreased motor skill efficiency)

- Sensory preferences (e.g., increased or decreased sensory sensitivities)

- Sensory and occupational deprivation

- Roles, relationships, feelings of self-worth and self-identity

- Participation in roles, routines, and activities (e.g., driving, household chores, leisure activities, work or volunteer activities, holiday celebrations)

There are times when symptoms that mimic those of dementia may arise, such as when people are feeling depressed, experiencing certain medication side effects, consuming alcohol excessively, experiencing significant hormonal changes, having vitamin deficiencies, or thyroid problems (*ibid.*). When symptoms of dementia occur for these reasons, it is typically reversible once the cause is identified and treated (*ibid.*).

Types of dementia

While many different types of dementia have been identified, Alzheimer's is the most common type, and it accounts for approximately 60–80 percent of all dementia cases. The second most common type of dementia is known as vascular dementia; this occurs when an individual experiences one or multiple infarcts (strokes) and residual brain damage, leading to cognitive decline and difficulty with other performance and participation skills (AA 2017a). Oftentimes people who have strokes have more than one, which can be of varying degrees of severity. Furthermore, people experiencing strokes may also have seizures, due to disruption to the neurophysiology of the brain, negatively influencing the electrical patterns of activity within the brain.

When working with people with dementia, one must be aware that there are many different types of dementia, which can occur at different ages and not only in older adulthood. The following list provides an introduction to the different types of dementia:

- Alzheimer's:

    - Caused by: deposits of the protein fragment beta-amyloid (plaques) and twisted strands of neurofibrillary tangles, creating nerve cell damage and death to brain tissue.
    - Symptoms include: progressive worsening of memory and ability to communicate and care for one's self and home. There are three stages of dementia (mild, moderate, severe) and the symptoms grow in severity with each stage. The three stages of dementia are outlined further, later on in this chapter.

- Vascular:

    - Caused by: stroke and other blood vessel problems.
    - Symptoms include: impaired judgment, difficulty with the ability to make decisions, plan, or organize thoughts.

- Lewy body:

    - Caused by: abnormal aggregations (or clumps) of the protein alpha-synuclein in the brain.
    - Symptoms include: memory loss and thinking problems that are similar to those of Alzheimer's. However, initial or early symptoms such as sleep disturbances, well-formed visual hallucinations, slowness in gait, balance problems, or Parkinsonian-like movement features are more likely.

- Frontotemporal:

    - Caused by: shrinkage of the nerve cells in the frontal (front) and temporal (side) lobes of the brain.
    - Symptoms include: difficulty with personality and behavior changes, and difficulty with language skills and movement that worsen over time.

- Parkinson's:

    - Caused by: alpha-synuclein clumps developing in the substantia nigra of the brain. These clumps cause the degeneration of nerve cells that produce the neurotransmitter known as dopamine.

- Symptoms include: problems with movement, which are the commonest early signs. If dementia develops, symptoms are often similar to the Lewy body dementia type. The person's face may become fixed or expressionless over time, despite how they are feeling. Depression is also common among people with Parkinson's.

- Creutzfeldt–Jakob:

  - Caused by: a rapidly fatal disease that sets into motion a misfolded prion protein causing a "domino effect" whereby the brain folds incorrectly and subsequently malfunctions.
  - Symptoms include: memory impairment, difficulty with physical coordination, and behavioral changes.

- Normal pressure hydrocephalus:

  - Caused by: a build up of fluid in the brain.
  - Symptoms include: difficulty walking, memory loss, and the inability to control urination.

- Huntington's:

  - Caused by: a genetic condition that manifests as abnormalities in brain protein.
  - Symptoms include: abnormal involuntary movements, severe decline in thinking and reasoning skills, irritability, depression, and other mood changes.

- Wernicke–Korsakoff:

  - Caused by (most typically): heavy and prolonged alcohol consumption and a severe deficiency of thiamine (vitamin B-1).
  - Symptoms include: severe memory problems, although other areas are less affected.

- Mixed: refers to having two or more types of dementia that are present at the same time (e.g., Alzheimer's and normal pressure hydrocephalus).

Stages of dementia

There is a great deal of information in the literature regarding the different stages of dementia. The stages of dementia refer to the way in which dementia progresses over time, and how the corresponding symptoms and behaviors are categorized. One of the most common ways in which the stages of dementia are described is in three stages: early, middle, and late (AA 2017a). The following list provides examples of dementia symptoms that are common at each stage:

- Early stage (mild cognitive impairment):
    - Still able to function independently
    - Some problems with word finding
    - Some problems with memory
    - Forgetting names and where things are placed
    - Increased difficulty with planning and organizing
    - Increased anxiety, irritability, and depression

- Middle stage (moderate cognitive impairment):
    - Difficulty remembering information about one's personal history
    - Struggles with orientation to time (date, seasons) and place (where one lives/one's location/one's phone number)
    - Needs help choosing proper clothing for changing seasons
    - At higher risk of wandering or getting lost
    - Sleep changes
    - Difficulty controlling bladder/bowels
    - Personality and behavior changes (suspiciousness, compulsions, moody, withdrawn, repetitive behaviors)
    - Repeating stories without awareness of the repetitions

- Late stage (severe cognitive impairment):
    - Hallucinations and delusions
    - Significant difficulty responding to own environment
    - Full-time, around-the-clock assistance required with daily personal care
    - Difficulty socializing and communicating/carrying on a conversation (finding words or articulating phrases)
    - Loss of awareness of recent experiences
    - Not recognizing one's surroundings
    - High levels of assistance required to perform daily activities and personal care
    - Changes in physical abilities, including the ability to walk, sit and, eventually, swallow

- Increased difficulty with sleep
- Increased vulnerability to infections, especially pneumonia
- Personality changes (increased anger, aggression, agitation, significant emotional distress)

In the earlier stages of dementia, people are often able to remain at home with the support of family and friends. As the symptoms of dementia progress, some are able to continue to live at home with increased home and community-based supports, but others may need to access higher levels of care (e.g., in independent living facilities, skilled nursing facilities). When the symptoms of dementia begin to worsen to the degree that more significant safety concerns and a higher level of support is needed, individuals often become residents of skilled nursing facilities or other caregiving institutions that are able to provide 24-hour supervision and care. When the symptoms of dementia become increasingly more severe, people may demonstrate unsafe, paranoid, or aggressive behaviors. During these times, nurturing, reassuring, and comforting interventions are necessary. In the later stages, dementia also impacts physical capacities such as the ability to walk, swallow food, and sit upright without support and supervision. Table 1.1 outlines changes that occur during the different stages of dementia.

As cognition and sensory acuity become increasingly impaired, people frequently rely on the sensory systems that are functioning more optimally to help make sense of experiences. For instance, when hearing is impaired the visual or other sensory systems may be more heavily relied upon.

Table 1.1 Stages of dementia

Dementia stage	Symptoms and behaviors
Early stage (mild)	• Forgetfulness and recent or short-term memory problems • May use strategies to cope or disguise memory problems • May have increased difficulty with concentration • Episodes of anxiety and depression may occur
Middle stage (moderate)	• Significant problems with memory (recognizing people, lapses of time) • Difficulty with self- and home care (dressing, cooking, money management, shopping, sleep) • Disinhibited or other problematic behaviors • Problems with visual and spatial skills • Difficulty with balance begins
Late stage (severe)	• Difficulty making simple decisions • Difficulty with communicating • Significantly decreased mobility, strength, balance, and coordination • Increased physical rigidity in movements and higher risk for falls • Difficulty with eating, swallowing, and with all self-care activities

Environmental sensory supportive cues that help each person feel oriented, safe, and able to participate in daily routines and activities are important.

Hallucinations, delusions, and paranoia

Hallucinations, delusions, and paranoia are common experiences for people in the mid to late stages of dementia. Problems with sensory acuity (hearing and visual problems) make identifying and interpreting sensations from the physical environment more challenging and can contribute to misinterpretations. Hallucinations, however, are false perceptions that are based on sensory experiences occurring without the presence of an external stimulus (AA 2017b; Teeple, Caplan, & Stern 2009). Changes in the brain contribute to the higher probability of experiencing hallucinations and delusions in people with dementia.

Delusions are thoughts that people perceive as real but are not accurate (AA 2017b). Believing that someone is being contacted one when it is not occurring is one example of a delusion that is not based in reality. Delusions may or may not be accompanied by paranoia. Suspiciousness is at the heart of paranoid thoughts and is common in people with dementia, such as thinking someone has stolen a possession when it has not happened. Hallucinations, delusions, and paranoid thoughts are not always upsetting to the person with dementia but at times can lead to severe upset, agitation, and aggression (AA 2017b). Certainly, having difficulty with memory, sensory processing, and the added experiences of hallucinations, delusions, or paranoia can make the world an overwhelming and scary place at times.

The stress response

The stress response is supported by the autonomic nervous system, which adjusts the functions of the body and one's level of autonomic arousal in response to experiences and perceptions. When a person is feeling overstimulated or overwhelmed, the stress response is triggered. Feeling stressed can occur for any number of reasons, and when a person is vulnerable and unable to modulate how they feel, this can lead to anxiety, agitation, and aggression. When people are more depressed or have the type of nervous system that requires more stimulation to process information, this can also lead to feelings of stress, anxiety, or trouble with attention span. One of the goals of using sensory approaches is to identify the individual's sensory processing patterns and corresponding sensory strategies and activities that will help to keep the stress response under control in order to support self-regulation and safety.

Working with people with dementia

For people who enjoy caring for others and spending time with older persons, working with people with dementia is highly rewarding! Whether caring for a loved one at home, in a community-based program, or skilled nursing facility, working with people with dementia can be fun, challenging, and deeply gratifying. While there will be many days when things will go smoothly, like in any area of practice, there will also be harder times. When people are struggling with memory problems, feelings of paranoia and restlessness, and possibly agitation, it is critical to have the training, tools, and supports necessary to both help them and maintain a safe and therapeutic environment. Having care practices in place that provide the means to help everyone feel comfortable, safe, and supported is key.

Recently, there have been a growing number of initiatives regarding the prevention of dementia and increasing the quality of care provided to people with dementia. These efforts to increase quality of care frequently spark a variety of state, national, and international initiatives. Organizations such as the Alzheimer's Association have websites offering a variety of resources, which demonstrate the different efforts taking place in research and the identification of the best and most promising practices.

Several different countries have focused significant resources on researching concerns related to certain practices with people with dementia, such as seclusion and restraint, which may include the overuse of antipsychotic medications (medicines are sometimes used as a form of chemical restraint) (Gitlin, Kales, & Lyketsos 2012; US Food and Drug Administration 2013). Several of these practices are used in the name of safety, but at times certain practices may be far from humane or therapeutic for those involved. In fact, both staff and clients are frequently injured when restraint or seclusion are used. The following sections review some of the recent initiatives related to these concerning practices with people with dementia. Sensory-based approaches and integrative frameworks, such as the Sensory Modulation Program (SMP), are therapeutic approaches that are useful in helping to decrease the use of restraint and overmedication. Sensory-based approaches that offer a range of options for the different senses, in a manner that is skilled and responsible, are increasingly used with people with dementia with positive effects, such as increased feelings of being calm, comforted, and nurtured (Champagne 2011; Klages *et al.* 2011). Sensory-based approaches are part of the movement to offer more non-pharmacological intervention options to people with dementia (Grasel, Wiltfang, & Kornhuber 2003; Hulme *et al.* 2010; Kong, Evans, & Guevara, 2009; Kverno *et al.* 2009; Robinson *et al.* 2007).

Restraint and seclusion reduction

Restraint and seclusion are sometimes used with people with dementia with the intention of keeping them safe (e.g., to decrease fall risk, to prevent the removal of a medical device, to stop harming one's self or others). A *restraint* is a chemical intervention (e.g., medication), physical method (e.g., physical hold), mechanical device (e.g., wrist restraint), or environmental barrier (e.g., tray tables, gates) used against one's will, which is not easily removed or avoided by the individual, and restricts freedom of movement or general access to one's own body or the bodies of others. *Seclusion* is the involuntary physical isolation of an individual, such as when a person is placed or locked in a room alone from which they cannot leave. The restraint and seclusion reduction initiative is part of a much larger, overarching, and international initiative to decrease the use of such violent and punitive interventions and to create a trauma-informed, comforting, and nurturing culture of care (National Executive Training Institute [NETI] 2003, 2009). The restraint and seclusion reduction initiative began with its application in mental healthcare settings but has expanded to include a variety of other populations and settings, such as those providing services to people with dementia (Champagne 2011). Sensory-based approaches are promoted as a way to help decrease the use of restraints and to increase the use of holistic, nurturing, and trauma-informed care practices (*ibid.*; Champagne & Stromberg 2004).

Trauma-informed care

Trauma-informed care refers to care that is "grounded in and directed by a thorough understanding of the neurological, biological, psychological and social effects of trauma and violence on humans and is informed by knowledge of the prevalence of these experiences in persons who receive services" (National Association of State Mental Health Program Directors [NASMHPD] 2000, p. 1). Trauma-informed care also requires that the care provided addresses trauma-related symptoms as part of the care delivery process and that care is collaborative and individualized to the person's specific needs and goals. Many people with dementia have trauma histories (e.g., war, domestic violence, medically-induced) and, therefore, it is essential to be aware of any trauma-related incidents, symptoms, triggers, or sensitivities an individual has or may have had at different points in their life. Furthermore, having dementia and experiencing the many ways in which it impacts one's life may be viewed by some as traumatic in and of itself.

For these reasons, trauma-informed care is an international initiative that also corresponds with dementia care.

In order to meet the charge of the restraint and seclusion reduction and trauma-informed care initiatives, it is necessary to identify and research innovative, promising, and evidence-based practices that support the ability to offer more nurturing and comforting interventions and environments of care. Healthcare providers are eagerly searching for such interventions to help prevent the use of restraint and seclusion. Sensory-based approaches are promoted as strategies that can be used to help decrease the use of restraint and seclusion (Champagne 2011; LeBel & Champagne 2010).

International initiatives in dementia care

The United States, Canada, Australia, and the United Kingdom all have national initiatives targeting the importance of non-pharmacological interventions and decreasing the use of restraint and seclusion with a variety of populations, including people with dementia. As part of the restraint and seclusion reduction initiative, there has been a concerted effort to decrease the use of antipsychotic medications with older persons with dementia. For instance, in Canada, the Canadian Foundation for Healthcare Improvement is instituting long-term care homes, and provincial–territorial government efforts include changing the culture of overmedicating seniors with dementia (see CFHI 2014). Overmedicating people with dementia is often used in the attempt to reduce aggressive or difficult behaviors. In accordance, the CFHI promotes increasing individualized, alternative, non-pharmacological behavioral support programs for people with dementia residing in long-term care facilities. In order to meet this charge, healthcare providers must obtain more comprehensive information on client histories, conduct regular medication reviews, and work as care teams with the client, family members, and previous caregivers, when appropriate. These efforts will ultimately help the staff working with people with dementia and their families tailor the services provided to support an increase in the quality of care and quality of life for residents. The skilled use of sensory approaches may assist organizations in reaching these goals, and ultimately most non-pharmacological interventions are sensory-based at their deepest core. Thus, the primary goal of using a more sensory-based approach is to be more strategic in its application, to provide the most individualized and helpful therapeutic plan for the person with dementia and involved family members.

Similar to the Canadian initiative, in 2013 the National Health and Medical Research Council in Australia launched a partnership focused on working with older persons with cognitive and related functional decline. This initiative gained momentum when it was identified that 9 percent of Australians over the age of 65 have some form of dementia and, therefore, the primary goal of this initiative is to create practice guidelines for working with people with dementia in community, hospital, and residential care settings (Laver *et al.* 2016).

The US and the UK are also working on initiatives related to the needs of people with dementia and have focused efforts and funding in similar ways to Canada and Australia. The US, for instance, launched a significant research initiative focusing on the identification of treatments that will prevent, and provide more effective treatment to those with Alzheimer's disease (US Department of Health and Human Services [USDHHS] 2013). The US has also passed legislation that increases access to innovative therapies and resources for people with dementia, including the implementation of *special care units* that provide some of the following (Reimer *et al.* 2004; Responsible Reform for the Middle Class 2010):

- Enhanced care through attention to both social and physical environments

- Medical care

- Meaningful activities

- Greater personal contact

One of the accomplishments in the UK is the development of a web-based resource providing care guidelines for a variety of disorders and diseases, including dementia (National Institute for Health and Care Excellence [NICE] 2017). (For more information on this web-based resource, refer to the Resources section at the end of the book.) Clearly, efforts have been made and are continuing to help find strategies for working with people with dementia that are more effective and humane.

Sensation is the primary gateway through which we perceive our experiences and communicate with others (Champagne 2017). Sensory strategies are promoted as an innovative and promising therapeutic approach that may help to reduce and prevent the use of restraint and seclusion (National Executive Training Institute 2003, 2009). The SMP provides a framework for planning and implementing the use of sensory-based strategies across systems of care and consumer populations (Champagne 2011; Champagne & Stromberg 2004).

When introducing the use of sensory-based strategies, the ability to identify which sensory strategies will be most impactful requires an individualized approach, including an assessment process focusing on sensory integration and processing. The ability to identify the client's sensory patterns and preferences supports the ability to collaboratively design individualized, therapeutic goals and plans. In situations where the client is not able to engage in the assessment process, authorized caregivers and family members may participate in the assessment process to help gather relevant information. Sensory approaches are also used to enhance the overall programming and physical environments of care settings providing services to people with dementia (inpatient units, day programs, long-term care).

The SMP is a general framework that outlines the programmatic components necessary to offer comprehensive, sensory-supportive approaches on individual and programmatic scales (Champagne 2011). In this way, the SMP provides resources that can be used to help family members, caregivers, organizations, and healthcare professionals in the effort to provide non-pharmacological interventions for people with dementia. Training by professionals skilled in sensory-based approaches is strongly recommended prior to the application of the SMP in the workplace. More information on the SMP is provided in Chapter 3.

Chapter 2

Aging and Sensory Processing

Sensation is energy or information that is detected by the specialized receptors (nerve endings) of the various sensory systems (eyes, ears, nose, mouth, skin, muscles, and joints). The ability to detect sensory stimuli is the first step in the process of taking in sensory-based information from the physical environment and from the body, and thereby integrating that information in order to make use of it. Sensory receptors are located in each of the sensory systems and play a significant role in how efficiently sensory stimuli are received and transmitted to the brain. Problems at the receptor level are usually referred to as issues with sensory acuity; however, these issues are not necessarily at deeper levels of sensory processing in the brain, such as when a person is near-sighted but wearing glasses enhances the ability to see things in the distance more clearly. Therefore, if the person has difficulty with sensory integration and processing, simply wearing glasses would not fully restore all visual abilities (e.g., visual perception). Thus, it is important to understand that there is a significant difference between the efficient detection of sensory stimuli (at the receptor level) and sensory integration and processing that take place within the brain. As people age, one, several, or even all of the sensory receptors may become less efficient due to deconditioning, injury, illness, or the aging process. Difficulty with processing sensory-based information beyond the level of sensory acuity is also common in people with dementia.

Once sensory input is received by the different sensory receptors and sent to the brainstem (located at the base of the brain), the nerve impulses then converge and diverge in the midbrain, sending the information to the higher cortical areas of the brain. At the higher cortical areas of the brain, the information is no longer in the form of "raw sensory data," and instead becomes integrated and informs one's larger perceptual experiences and awareness of one's self in the world. Sensation also has a significant influence on perception. Perception is the process by which the brain selects, organizes, and interprets all sensation (energy or information) (Freeman 2000). Sensory integration and processing are terms that are often used interchangeably when referring to the nervous system processing that occurs beyond the receptor level of sensory acuity. When dementia occurs it targets the brain and, therefore, it impacts sensory integration and processing as well. Since dementia typically occurs later in life, many people will have problems with various aspects of sensory acuity (receptor level) as well as sensory integration and processing (higher level processing that occurs in the brain).

People of all ages and abilities need daily, sensory-rich experiences because sensation provides nourishment for the nervous system (Ayres 1979). Sensory supportive experiences help foster feelings of safety and orientation, and the ability to engage in relationships, roles, routines, and activities. Individuals with dementia are frequently dependent upon caregivers to help them engage in comfortable, active, sensory-rich experiences that have been individually tailored to their needs, and caregivers also help to ensure that environments of care are humane, safe, and holistic. The ability to provide sensory-rich experiences safely and skillfully requires an understanding of: (1) the sensory systems, (2) how the brain works to integrate and process sensory-related information, (3) safety considerations, (4) how aging and dementia play a role, and (5) what the Sensory Modulation Program encompasses.

The sensory systems and aging

Many people are aware of the five basic sensory systems; however, there are actually eight sensory systems: proprioception, vestibular, tactile, vision, auditory, olfactory, gustatory, and interoception. Understanding the unique contribution of each of the sensory systems is important. Such an understanding will contribute to the ability to realize how each of the sensory systems plays a role in supporting function and quality of life.

Additionally, the ability to create sensory supportive interventions requires an understanding of how to use different types of sensory input to support a variety of therapeutic goals. For example, if a person is having difficulty with body awareness, identifying and providing activities or modalities that are enjoyable and rich in tactile and proprioceptive input may help the person feel more bodily aware (e.g., having a manicure, petting a dog, sorting different types of fabric, using a weighted lap pad).

Proprioceptive system: sense of bodily awareness, body position, and movement

Have you ever wondered how you are able to feel grounded in your body and anchored in the world—without having to even think about it? What would it be like to not have this ability or if it became increasingly difficult to feel self-aware? Proprioception is a form of sensory input that contributes to bodily awareness and the ability to know where one's body is in space and time, from a body-based "felt" sense. The sensory receptors of the proprioceptive system are sometimes referred to as proprioceptors. Proprioceptors are the receptors of the proprioceptive system that are located in the muscles, ligaments, tendons, joints, connective tissues, and fascia—throughout the entire body. You can think of your muscles as major sensory organs. When people are not active for any number of reasons, immobility and deconditioning impact the ability of the proprioceptive system to operate efficiently.

Occasionally with aging, the amount of muscle tissue and strength a person has decreases due to limitations in mobility as a result of experiencing pain (e.g., arthritis), injury (e.g., fractures), becoming less active (deconditioning), and because the hormones that support muscle growth tend to decrease with age, and any number of degenerative disorders (Levin 2016). Additionally, a host of other neurophysiological changes may occur with aging, further contributing to possible deconditioning, weakness, and muscle atrophy (wasting away of muscle tissue) (Campellone 2016; Levin 2016). Those with muscle atrophy, due to the lack of movement, can be helped to regenerate muscle tissue and strength through daily opportunities for preferred types of active movement, exercise, and nutrition (Campellone 2016). People with dementia sometimes remain sedentary (in seated or lying down positions), may experience being physically restrained for periods of time, and may even become chair- or bedridden—all of which can contribute to the development of weakness, muscle atrophy, and problems with proprioception and body awareness. Thus, it is critical to provide safe, supportive, and daily means for active movement to prevent, and in some cases reverse, muscle weakness, atrophy, and even contractures (stiffening and deformity of joints).

Active engagement in stretching and different kinds of movement, preferably through purposeful activities, is critical to sustaining strength, flexibility, and range of motion. At the same time, given the wide range of other physical and medical limitations a person may have (e.g., cardiac, respiratory, arthritis, fragile skin), it is essential to work with doctors and rehabilitation professionals to identify the safest and most appropriate movement-based activities, stretches, exercises, and safety precautions to use with each individual. There is a significant amount of research supporting the positive effects of exercise and yoga (modified as needed) for people with dementia (Fan & Chen 2011; Lee, Park, & Park 2016; Oken *et al.* 2006). An individualized routine can be provided by a rehabilitation professional that is safe and tailored to the person's therapeutic needs, goals, and safety concerns. Sensory-based activities that offer increased proprioceptive input can provide the additional input people need to feel more grounded in their bodies, safe, and more oriented. Chapter 5 offers examples of different activities and modalities that provide an increase in proprioceptive input to the body.

The proprioceptive system does not operate in isolation. It is highly interconnected with the tactile and vestibular systems in order to help provide a complex, coherent, and organized sense of self in space and time. Thus, when engaging in activities that influence the proprioceptive system, these other sensory systems are also influenced.

Vestibular system: sense of space, balance, and movement

The vestibular system is located in the inner ear mechanism on both sides of the head and is stimulated during movement of the head and body. The vestibular system consists of the semicircular canals and the otoliths. The semicircular canals detect rotation and angular movements (arcs). The otoliths detect gravity and linear movements, and include the utricle and saccule. The utricle picks up on horizontal (linear) movements and the saccule picks up on vertical (linear) movements.

The vestibular system functions similarly to that of a GPS (global positioning system), in that it helps to provide a gravitational reference point from which we detect movement (spatial awareness, directionality, balance) and speed (e.g., acceleration, deceleration, timing). Specifically, the vestibular system contributes to the sense of balance/equilibrium, spatial awareness, extensor (muscle) tone, and postural control, and supports the coordination, efficiency, and fluidity of movements.

The vestibular system is also interconnected with the auditory, visual, and proprioceptive systems. These sensory systems work together to support an oriented, coherent, and safe experience of the world. When any one or more of these sensory systems is not operating optimally, the person may be fearful and anxious, and experience difficulty with everyday functioning. When coupling difficulty with sensory processing and trouble with cognitive functioning due to dementia, it becomes easy to understand why a sensory supportive approach is essential.

Balance

One of the primary areas of concern when caring for a person with dementia, related to the vestibular system, is balance. Changes in balance increase the risk of falling. Balance refers to the ability to maintain the body's central reference point and body positioning against gravity. When the sensory systems supporting balance are functioning well, people are able to see clearly, easily orient themselves in and through space, make automatic postural adjustments, and remain stable as they move and ambulate (Vestibular Disorders Association 2017). In order to support balance, the vestibular, proprioceptive, tactile, and visual systems work together to process the multisensory input involved. More simply put, stimulation received from the eyes, vestibular organs, and muscles and joints work together to support balance (*ibid.*). The cerebellum is part of the brain that also works with these sensory systems to support movement and balance (*ibid.*). The sensorimotor input is processed and integrated through the lower to the higher centers of the brain, and the result of that continuous, dynamic process is evident in how well the person is able to move and ambulate (walk) in the environment. As people age, and certainly when people have neurodegenerative diseases such as dementia, progressive difficulty with balance, irregularity in gait (walking), dizziness, and problems with coordination, movement, and increased falls are more common. Figure 2.1 demonstrates how these sensory systems work in conjunction with the cerebellum (sensorimotor input) to support balance (sensorimotor output).

According to El-Khoury *et al.* (2013), exercise helps to decrease falls and injuries caused by falling. Multisensory environments can be used to foster movement and improved balance (Klages *et al.* 2011). Skilled rehabilitation services and daily movement opportunities that do not overstimulate, overwhelm, or cause discomfort or harm to the individual can assist the maintenance of functional skills and quality of life for as long as possible. For some individuals, depending upon the type of vestibular disorder(s) experienced, vestibular rehabilitation services may also help.

Before or during the progression of dementia, it is possible that other problems may manifest that can lead to issues with balance and eye coordination, and increasing symptoms of dizziness or vertigo. This is not an all-inclusive list, but some examples of other vestibular disorders include:

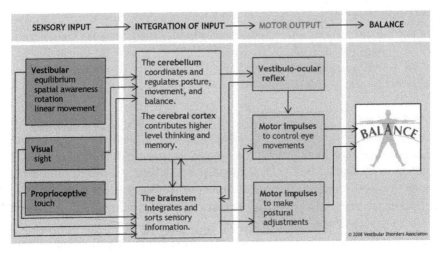

Figure 2.1 The human balance system
Source: Reproduced with the permission of the Vestibular Disorders Association (2017).

- Acoustic neuroma
- Autoimmune inner ear disease
- Benign paroxysmal vertigo
- Bilateral vestibular hypofunction
- Canvas syndrome
- Cervicogenic dizziness
- Concussion
- Enlarged vestibular aqueduct syndrome
- Labyrinthitis and vestibular neuritis
- Ménière's disease
- Neurotoxicity
- Ototoxicity
- Perilymph fistula
- Persistent postural perceptual dizziness
- Tinnitus
- Vestibular hyperacusis

- Vestibular insufficiency

When a sudden change occurs in a person's balance or there is a sudden onset of symptoms of dizziness or vertigo, assessment by a rehabilitation professional skilled in vestibular rehabilitation may be helpful to diagnose the cause of the problem and identify potential avenues of treatment.

Psychosocial considerations

People experiencing difficulty with processing vestibular stimulation frequently become very anxious, agitated, or even assaultive when they are moved suddenly or feel unsafe during movement or self-care management. It is paramount to acknowledge that, when experiencing all of the different symptoms of dementia, and compounding those symptoms with difficulty in vestibular processing, it is vital to identify ways in which to help the person feel safe, comfortable, and supported during all movements and activities.

Finding ways in which to help them feel safe during activities requiring movement or when being moved or touched is one means of assisting those whose vestibular functioning is impaired. Useful approaches include helping clients to feel securely held and safe, offering reassurance, helping them to feel oriented, encouraging them to be an active participant in what is happening as much as possible, and refocusing their attention when necessary. There are a variety of sensory tools that can help. Comforting sensations, using a supportive tone of voice, approaching from within the person's visual field (front), moving slowly and not abruptly, making sure the person is not too cold or too warm, and having something secure to hold are just a few sensory-based strategies that can help.

The benefits derived from the use of sensory strategies that offer comforting forms of vestibular stimulation in a safe and skilled way are not limited to those who have difficulty with vestibular processing. Sensory strategies that offer vestibular input in a manner that may be perceived as helpful for some individuals include: rocking or gliding in a rocker, exercises or stretching performed from a seated position, games that require reaching (balloon volleyball), swaying to preferred forms of music, and many more! These strategies can be used to help the person feel safe, calm, and more attentive and oriented, and can be used to help decrease deconditioning (when safe and appropriate). For more sensory-based, vestibular strategy examples and corresponding information regarding safety and vestibular stimulation, refer to Chapter 5.

Visual system: sense of sight

The visual system is the most complex of all sensory systems and aids individuals in the tasks of seeing, looking, and focusing on visual stimuli (reading, looking at a photograph album, looking into a family member's eyes). The visual system concurrently contributes to the sense of spatial awareness, balance, and equilibrium because it is interconnected with the vestibular system.

Many people experience changes in visual acuity and visual perception with age. A few of these changes include the decreased flexibility of the eye musculature, impacting the ability to achieve full range of motion with both eyes, which may also contribute to difficulty with peripheral vision, visual scanning, and tracking (e.g., looking in different directions without having to move one's head). Trouble with depth perception makes it harder to discern the foreground from the background, impacting the ability to perform functional tasks. For example, finding something in a crowded drawer or estimating the depth of a step when stepping down from a curb requires depth perception. As people age, there is often decreased sensitivity of the cornea, leading to increased potential for eye injuries to go unnoticed (Martin 2016). Pupils decrease in size by approximately one-third and respond to changes in light less efficiently. The lens of the eye may thicken and become less flexible, cloudy, and yellowed, making it more challenging to see clearly. There is frequently increased difficulty with the ability to detect contrasts in the environment and increased sensitivity to extreme changes in lighting (brightness, glare, darkness). Reduced ability to recognize objects and detect colors, and issues with double vision are also possible as people age. There are a variety of diseases that negatively impact the vision of older persons. These include but are not limited to: cataracts, glaucoma, macular degeneration, diabetic retinopathy, hypertensive retinopathy, temporal arteritis, and detached retina (Cacchione 2017; Martin 2016).

Approximately 30 percent of people over the age of 65 will become visually impaired (visual acuity of 20/50 or worse), legally blind (20/200 or worse as best corrected vision), or totally blind (no light perception) (Cacchione 2017). Given that the visual field narrows as dementia progresses, it is necessary to place desired items or objects within the person's visual field (Allen, Earhart, & Blue 1999). A research study by Brush and Caulkins (2008) revealed that some of the significant environmental stressors of older persons include: visual overstimulation, difficulty with visual contrast, and different types of and changes in lighting, glare, and auditory confusion. In accordance, reducing visual chaos, clutter, and glare in the environment is recommended when working with people with dementia (Caspari, Eriksson, & Nåden 2011). Providing adequate lighting and visual contrasts in the environment and during self-care activities is necessary; for example, having highly contrasting colors between the table (or tablecloth), plate, cup, and utensils to support ease in distinguishing each item from the background of the table (or tablecloth). It is important to schedule regular eye care visits, to ensure the individual wears eye glasses as prescribed, and to obtain treatment for any problems related to visual health. Visual screenings can also become increasingly complicated as dementia progresses, as many visual screenings rely on accurate reporting; nevertheless, the ability to provide proper visual supports and eye care is critical across the lifespan.

Visual hallucinations may be present as part of the symptomatology of many different disorders, including dementia. When visual hallucinations are present in a person in the early to middle phases of dementia, it may lead to the identification of Lewy body dementia (Teeple *et al.* 2009). It is imperative to work with a physician to identify the cause of hallucinations when they occur in order to determine the dementia type and thus the most effective form(s) of treatment. Additionally, helping to assess the situation and distinguish between visual hallucinations versus misperceptions or misidentifications is also important; for instance, dark-colored flooring may look like a deep hole, or glare from natural lighting may cause visual distortions that could seem like hallucinations if not fully assessed (AA 2017b).

Providing reassurance, support, distractions, and other non-pharmacological interventions, such as individualized sensory approaches, are helpful in calming and comforting the person experiencing visual hallucinations, distortions, or misperceptions. Environmental modifications are also part of the SMP, and some examples of environmental modifications include: using contrasting colors (highlighting important items, reducing attention to certain areas [exit doors]), being attentive to the décor in the environment, providing even, adequate lighting throughout the setting to prevent shadows and visual distortions, and closing the windows and curtains at night. These adaptations to the environment are some of the proactive ways in which to support the person with dementia from needless fears and worries.

The various changes in visual processing, when coupled with other symptoms of dementia—such as fear, anxiety, disorientation, paranoia, and hallucinations—contribute to increased risk for falls, a more sedentary lifestyle, and decreased participation in roles and activities. In addition to those explored, several sensory strategies can be used to support people experiencing problems with visual processing and dementia, including those that provide appropriate forms of visual stimulation when individualized to the person's needs and preferences. Refer to Chapter 5 for more examples of different sensory strategies that can be helpful.

Auditory system: sense of sound

The ability to hear, listen, locate the directionality of sound(s), and distinguish between differences in loudness, pitch, and timbre is reliant upon the efficient functioning of the auditory system. In order to understand more about the structure and function of the auditory system, a brief review of the anatomy of the ear and how an auditory stimulus supports the ability to hear is provided.

The structures of the auditory system reside in the areas of the outer ear, middle ear, and inner ear. The outer ear is the part of the ear that is seen on each side of the head (called the pinnae), and includes the auditory canal leading to the middle ear. The middle ear is located inside of the head, and houses the tiny bones, ligaments, membranes, muscles, hair cells, and fluids that support the functioning of the auditory system. The outer ear helps capture sound waves and guide them into the auditory canal. Once in the canal, the sound waves will encounter the eardrum (tympanic membrane), which protects the middle ear. The eardrum not only protects the middle ear but also turns sound waves into vibrations that are projected into the middle ear.

The bones of the middle ear are said to be the smallest bones of the body, and are called the malleus, incus, and stapes. These three bones transmit the vibrations from the eardrum to the membrane that covers the oval window. From the point of the oval window, the vibrations are transmitted to the cochlea (snail-like, bony structure), contained within the inner ear. The cochlea is fluid-filled and contains inner and outer hair cells. The inner and outer hair cells have cilia that extend out beyond the hair cells. Vibration of the cilia causes them to bend, which generates an electrical signal that releases a neurotransmitter, which then sends a signal to the brain through the auditory nerve.

Many people acknowledge how important it is to be able to hear, and the role that hearing plays in the ability to communicate; however, most do not understand that the auditory system also supports the ability to self-regulate. Consider how listening to your favorite music can lift your mood and how other types of music you might listen to make you want to rest or calm you. Furthermore, the sense of sound may serve as a mode of protection, such as when hearing the sound of an alarm, someone screaming for help, or other sounds that are meant to grab your attention. What many people do not realize is that the auditory system also helps people feel organized, supports the ability to pay attention, helps people recognize sense of rhythm and timing, and assists in the ability to speak.

Presbycusis is the term used to describe the age-related changes that impact the ability to hear, which typically occurs in both ears. Interestingly, the third most common condition in people over the age of 75 is hearing loss (Cacchione 2017). This decline in the ability to hear simultaneously creates issues with localizing sound (the ability to know where different sounds are coming from). Other types of hearing loss are due to ear infections, meningitis, trauma to the auditory system (e.g., nerve damage), and a variety of other reasons that may affect one or both ears. Hearing loss makes hearing people talk or listening to different sounds arduous, particularly when there is competing noise (e.g., background noise). The ability to hear someone talk when using a telephone, during social groups and gatherings, or when music or the television is playing can be strenuous and frustrating as a result of hearing loss. Hearing aids are commonly provided to those with hearing loss to help compensate, but not all types of hearing loss respond well to them (e.g., nerve damage).

Problems with auditory discrimination refer to having an auditory processing complication that is not caused by issues at the level of the auditory receptor(s) (acuity), and, therefore, it is frequently referred to as an auditory processing disorder or auditory discrimination problem. In people with an auditory processing disorder, the complications are caused by a central nervous system processing issue. When difficulties related to an auditory processing disorder occur, hearing aids will not be effective or even prescribed. Nevertheless, the individual with auditory processing problems will have trouble with different aspects of hearing or attention difficulties, and may struggle with listening (National Coalition of Auditory Processing Disorders 2017). While many people often think of an auditory processing disorder as a problem typically seen in children, when left unattended it may continue into adulthood.

Another factor that impacts auditory processing capacity is being in a stressful or fearful state. The autonomic nervous system prioritizes safety. When the fight, flight, or freeze response is triggered it can lead to a gradual or sudden shutdown in the ability to process auditory information. Helping the person feel safe and secure can ease this autonomic nervous system response and change the ability to receive and process auditory information, thereby making it easier to hear and communicate.

There are multiple ways in which to use sound to help people with dementia feel more attentive, comforted, regulated, and able to increase participation in daily life activities. A variety of sensory strategies related to the sense of sound will be covered in Chapter 5.

Gustatory system: sense of taste

The gustatory system refers to the sense of taste. The sense of taste is primarily supported by the chemical receptors of the tongue known as the taste buds. Each taste bud detects a different type of taste sensation, such as sweet, sour, salty, bitter, and savory. There are other sensory systems that support the functioning of the mouth and jaw, such as the tactile and proprioceptive systems. The tactile receptors of the mouth detect the temperature and textures of foods, vibration, and pain. The muscles and joints of the mouth and jaw aid in the coordination of sipping, drinking, chewing, swallowing, blowing, and speaking.

Difficulties with the sense of taste frequently happen at the receptor level (taste buds) but may also occur at a higher level of sensory integration and processing as well. Adults have approximately 5000–9000 taste buds. Not only does this number reduce with age, but the taste buds also begin decreasing in sensitivity after the age of 60 (Cacchione 2017; Lane, Smith Roley, & Champagne 2014). Taste discrimination impacts the ability to differentiate between various tastes, enjoy the tastes of foods, drink fluids, and perform activities of daily living, such as eating and teeth brushing. Moreover, as dementia progresses, the ability to coordinate the muscles of the mouth to support the safe and functional ability to drink, chew, and swallow is gradually impacted. A variety of sensory strategies related to the sense of taste and oral motor input will be covered in Chapter 5.

Olfactory system: sense of smell

The sense of smell is dependent upon the chemical receptors of the nose and can be thought of as a chemical reaction. The senses of smell and taste work together to help us enjoy what we smell, eat, and drink. The sensory receptors of the nose are located in the upper section of the nasal cavity, and detect chemicals known to most people as scents. The olfactory receptors project olfactory stimuli to the olfactory bulb, and from that point to the olfactory tracts. The olfactory tracts bring the olfactory information deep into the brain, to the limbic system (emotion center of the brain). The effects of smelling something are almost instantaneous, because the messages travel from the receptors of the nose to the brain at a speed of approximately 300 miles per hour!

The olfactory system is one of the few sensory systems that directly projects to the emotion and memory centers of the brain. This is why certain scents can lead to a fairly quick emotional response and may trigger memories (positive or negative in nature). Therefore it is crucial to be cautious with the types and intensity of scents used with people, and to understand that a person with dementia may be triggered by scents in a way that may or may not be easily understood or described.

The processes of aging and dementia often cause the olfactory receptors to function inefficiently, leading to trouble discerning between different types of scent. With aging there is frequently a decrease in the production of mucous in the nose, also diminishing the ability to retain odors to support the process of olfaction. Whether or not an individual has issues with olfaction, the use of scents can be a very positive and supportive sensory-based intervention. The ability to provide scents that are perceived as supportive and comforting to the person can be highly therapeutic. For a list of sensory-based options related to the sense of smell, refer to Chapter 5.

Tactile system: sense of touch

There are several distinct receptors in the skin that contribute to the sense of touch, usually referred to as the tactile system. The tactile system is the largest of the sensory systems because the tactile receptors are located in the skin, which is the body's container. Many people think of the tactile system simplistically, but it is actually very complex. There are six types of touch receptors that detect particular types of touch sensation:

1. Free nerve endings: detect pain, temperature, and touch

2. Merkel's disk: detects light pressure and perceives fine differences

3. Perifollicular: detects when body or face is touched (wrap-around hair follicles)

4. Ruffini corpuscles: detect touch pressure and stretch of the skin (have both tactile and proprioceptive roles)

5. Meissner's corpuscles: detect discrimination

6. Pacinian corpuscles: detect pressure and vibration

Touch stimuli ascend through the spinal cord and brainstem, cross midline (activating the thalamus on the opposite side of the stimulus), and continue to the primary sensory cortex in the postcentral gyrus of the brain.

Research has identified that therapeutic approaches providing pleasing forms of tactile stimulation increase task participation and decrease agitation (King 2012). Similar to the other sensory systems, the aging process can impact the ability to efficiently register different touch sensations. Additionally, as the severity of dementia progresses, problems with tactile processing may impact the ability to be aware of distinct tactile sensations. Some of the corresponding behaviors you may see include:

- Difficulty distinguishing, comparing, and contrasting

- Trouble detecting/being aware of temperature, pain, and vibration

- Difficulty localizing tactile input

- Inefficient hand manipulation skills (using utensils, pen/pencil, work tools) and handwriting

- Clumsiness

- Difficulty with body scheme/awareness

- Trouble with bodily boundaries (e.g., space invader, clingy, touches everything)

- Seems unaware of touch unless intense or seen visually

- Poor body awareness

- Oral motor and speech difficulties

- Sloppy eater; chews on things

- May hurt people/animals by using too much force without awareness

- Difficulty with stereognosis (identifying objects through touch without the use of vision)

Providing opportunities to explore different types of pleasant, tactile experiences specific to the person's needs may provide the input necessary to support tactile discrimination abilities as people age. For instance, folding activities offering a wide range of fabric textures, cooking activities (kneading dough, putting sprinkles on cookies), polishing silverware, going outdoors to experience different temperatures, and craft activities with a variety of safe materials rich in tactile input are all different examples of how to add a variety of tactile sensory-rich opportunities.

Some individuals may feel bothered by certain types of tactile stimulation with aging (cold temperatures, certain forms of touch, certain types of craft supplies [glue, paint]). Different types of tactile or touch sensitivities may appear or increase in people with dementia. It is paramount to assess the person's sensory preferences (likes and dislikes) before offering tactile or other sensory stimulation, in order to decrease the possibility of upsetting an individual with stimulation that may be bothersome. See Chapter 4 for more information on assessment.

Hyper-sensitivity (over-responsivity) to tactile stimulation may be due to changes in the skin of older adults impacting tactile receptors, skin tears or sores, or a history of tactile hyper-sensitivity that continues or worsens in older adulthood. Tactile hyper-sensitivity may influence an increase in the following behaviors and tendencies:

- Fight or flight response to touch (fearful response)

- Not liking to be touched

- Not liking messy foods or art activities

- Not liking self-care tasks (hair brushing)

- Not liking being located close to other people (sitting near someone, standing in lines, being in crowded spaces)

The decreased awareness of tactile sensation is often referred to as tactile hypo-sensitivity (under-responsivity), meaning that the person has less awareness of tactile sensations. For instance, when tactile hypo-sensitivity (under-responsivity) occurs, there is often a lack of awareness or slowed response to being touched, decreased pain awareness, less awareness of temperatures (water in the shower, temperature of a cup of tea, temperature in the home), clumsiness or difficulty with manipulating containers, fasteners, foods, craft supplies, and so on. While we have focused more on the possibility of having tactile hyper- or hypo-sensitivity patterns (over- or under-responsivity), it is possible to have these patterns in each of the sensory systems, thus demonstrating the complexity of sensory integration and processing and the importance of assessment in order to create skilled, comprehensive, and individualized therapeutic recommendations.

According to Chillot (2013), touch is commonly reported as one of the best ways to provide comfort (hugs, hand-holding, pats). There are many ways in which to provide tactile input that helps people with dementia feel more safe, comforted, and secure. Refer to Chapter 5 for a list of sensory-based strategies that may be used to provide more options for various types of tactile input.

Interoception: sense of internal self-awareness

The ability to be aware of whether you are tired, alert, hungry, in pain, not feeling well, and a host of other internal states or feelings within the body is referred to as interoception (Mahler 2017). Over time, having dementia causes difficulty with interoceptive capacities and the ability to communicate. Increased confusion and issues with changes in the brain and sensory systems with aging contribute to increased difficulty with interoceptive awareness. The following list provides examples of some that correspond with interoception, such as the ability to be aware of:

- Degree of sleepiness
- Degree of alertness
- Degree of pain
- Degree of thirst
- Degree of hunger
- Heart rate
- Pulse rate
- Body temperature
- Muscle tension
- Nausea
- Bowel and bladder sensations
- Detection of illness

When the stress response is triggered, several of the internal organs change the way in which they are functioning in order to mobilize the body to deal with the stressor or protect itself. Similarly, when calm, the bodily functions and emotional states adjust accordingly. The bodily and emotional states influence each other and alert us to safety concerns, comfort sensations, triggers, needs, and related emotions and behaviors. When a person anticipates a particular feeling and then perceives the related bodily sensations, the urge to act in relation to those feelings and sensations commonly follows (*ibid.*). Furthermore, the impulse to act on an urge or inhibit the urge and the ability to self-regulate are interrelated. The more coherent the awareness of one's internal states, emotions, and urges, the more possibility there is for learning how to get one's needs met and to inhibit urges when needed. Interoceptive awareness is foundational to the ability to understand not only one's own personal inner states and needs, but also the potential states, needs, and perspectives of others (*ibid.*). In people with dementia, a coherent sense of self-awareness diminishes over time, impacting interoceptive awareness, impulse control, and the ability to self-regulate.

A general summary of each of the sensory systems and their corresponding sensory receptors and examples of some of the functional contributions of each of the sensory systems are provided in Table 2.1 (Champagne 2017).

In summary, the different sensory systems provide a gateway to fostering orientation, attention, feelings of safety and comfort, enhanced participation, and quality of life. The nervous system is continuously processing input from all of the sensory systems to produce a coherent, multisensory experience over time. Each person's perceptual representation of what they experience is unique. This knowledge supports the importance of using a sensory lens when working with people with dementia, to help identify and provide the customary type and amount of sensory input that people need for a variety of therapeutic reasons.

As people age, the ability to process sensory and motor stimulation from each of the various sensory systems is frequently negatively impacted for a variety of reasons (e.g., trauma, cognitive decline, injury, illness, neuropathies, spinal cord compression, brain lesions, neurodegenerative disease). When this occurs, active, engaging, sensory-rich activities and physical environments are particularly important, because sensory and motor capacities (e.g., eyesight, hearing, sense of taste, body awareness, balance) often diminish. Similar to the saying, "use it or lose it," it is important to think of sensory- and movement-based therapeutic interventions as a way to decrease or prevent the possibility of deconditioning and sensory deprivation. Sensory strategies may be used to help decrease agitation and the effects of sun downing, and to support active engagement in daily routines and activities (Doble & Vania 2009; King 2012).

Table 2.1 Sensory systems

Sensory systems and receptors	Primary function(s)	Contributions
Proprioception Receptors are located in the muscles, joints, ligaments, tendons, connective tissues, and fascia (e.g., muscle spindles, joint receptors, and golgi tendon organs). Receptors are stimulated by movements causing muscles to stretch, contract, or co-contract (particularly when movement is against resistance).	The proprioceptive system supports: body awareness, the ability to assume and maintain body positions, and the grading, timing, and efficiency of movements. The proprioceptive system works with the tactile system to support body awareness (body-based felt sense) and the vestibular system to support efficient and fluid movements and postural control (body in space).	Contributes to the awareness of: • Where the body and body parts are located in space and over time • Body movement • Body position • Body boundaries • Body image • Proprioceptive information from the environment providing safety-related cues
Vestibular The vestibular system structures are housed within the inner ear and include the otoliths (utricle and saccule) and semicircular canals. Receptors include tiny hair cells that bend with the movement of the fluid within the semicircular canals or by the shifting of the membrane into which the hairs cells project into the otoliths. Receptors (hair cells) are activated during acceleration, deceleration, spinning, linear, angular movements, any other movements involving the head, and the pull of gravity.	The vestibular system supports the ability to be aware of the spatial orientation of the body (including equilibrium, speed, timing, and rhythmicity of positioning and movement). The vestibular system works with the proprioceptive system to support efficient and fluid movements and postural control and the visual system to support the ability to maintain a stable visual field, balance, and equilibrium. The vestibular and auditory systems are also interconnected.	Contributes to: • Spatial awareness of where the body is in space and time • Balance • Body coordination • Muscle tone • Gravity detection • Awareness of the speed and direction of movements • Awareness of whether things around us are moving or stationary • Vestibular information from the environment providing safety-related cues

Tactile	The tactile system supports the ability to detect safety, comfort, and discomfort/pain (protective function), and to discriminate and localize stimulation detected by the tactile receptors.	Contributes to the awareness of:
Receptors are located in the skin (most dense in the hand, mouth, and genital areas).		• Tactile sensations and tactile discrimination
		• Pressure sensations (light/deep)
Receptors are activated during any type of skin contact (e.g., when touching something, showering, tooth brushing, eating, drinking, grooming, dressing).	The tactile system works with the proprioceptive system to support body awareness.	• Pain coming from the pain receptors of the skin
		• Temperature
		• Vibration
		• Body boundaries
		• Tactile information from the environment providing safety-related cues
Visual	The visual system supports the ability to discriminate visual stimuli in order to see, identify, and locate objects, symbols, boundaries, and people, and to map spatial relationships, etc.	Contributes to the awareness of:
Receptors are located in the retina of the eye (rods and cones) and stimulated by visual input (light, colors, contours, shades, etc.)		• Gradations of colors, lightness, darkness
		• Shapes, symbols, contours
		• Movement detection
	The visual system also works with the vestibular system to support a stable visual field, and supports balance and equilibrium.	• Visual information from the environment providing safety-related cues
Auditory	The auditory system supports the ability to detect the distance, directionality, and qualities of sounds.	Contributes to the awareness of:
The auditory receptors are the hair cells of the cochlea located within the inner ear and stimulated by sound waves and vibrations.		• Volume of sound(s)
	The auditory system is interconnected with the vestibular system.	• Tone of sound(s)
		• Directionality of sound(s)
Olfaction	The olfactory system supports the ability to detect and localize odors/scents, has a protective function, and has a direct connection to the limbic system (emotion center of the brain) to influence emotions.	Contributes to the awareness of:
The olfactory epithelium contains the chemical receptors of the nose, also called an osmoreceptor. The olfactory sense is stimulated by different scents.		• The nature of odors (pleasant, familiar, unpleasant)
		• How strong an odor is perceived to be
	The olfactory and gustatory systems work together to enhance the sense of taste.	• Olfactory information from the environment providing safety-related cues

(continued)

Sensory systems and receptors	Primary function(s)	Contributions
Gustatory Taste buds contain the chemical receptors of the tongue and are stimulated when tasting or manipulating things in the mouth (drinking, tasting, chewing).	The gustatory system assists in the ability to discriminate between different tastes and helps to gather information about stimuli entering the mouth. The gustatory and olfactory systems work together to enhance the sense of taste.	Contributes to the awareness of: • The nature of taste sensations (pleasant, familiar, unpleasant) • How strong the taste stimuli is perceived to be • Gustatory information from the environment providing safety-related cues
Interoception Sensory nerve endings contained within the muscles, organs, and viscera across the different systems within the body.	Interoception supports the ability to be aware of internal states and corresponding feelings, urges, and emotions.	Contributes to the awareness of: • Temperature • Pain • Hunger • Muscle tension • Sleepiness/alertness • Heart rate • Respiration rate • Digestion • Bowel/bladder functions • Nausea • Nervousness

Source: Reproduced with the permission of Champagne (2017).

As explored throughout this chapter, sensory-based approaches may be used for a variety of therapeutic purposes, including:

- Fostering safety (de-escalation and prevention)
- Fostering self-organization and self-regulation
- Shifting levels of alertness
- Providing compensatory supports
- Providing preparatory supports
- Providing nurturance and comfort
- Providing positive forms of distraction
- Promoting health, wellness, and quality of life
- Promoting participation (activities, routines, roles)

An individualized and skilled approach is key to identifying and providing the "just right" amount and type of daily, sensory-rich experiences, and activities to people with dementia.

Sensory integration and processing

There are many different schools of thought, theories, and terminology used to explain and research sensory integration and processing. While many of these terms will be explored in this section, one of the pioneers of sensory integration is Dr. A. Jean Ayres. Ayres (1972) defines sensory integration as "the neurological process that organizes sensation from one's body and from the environment and makes it possible to use the body efficiently within the environment" (p. 11).

Initially, Ayres created the framework and theory of sensory integration for working with children with a variety of learning and neurodevelopmental challenges. Over time, Ayres' work grew in its application to include both child and adult populations with a variety of distinct therapeutic needs and disorders. Ayres' sensory integration is often the body of work that many occupational therapists and other professionals reference to create other sensory-based models and interventions (Ayres 1989, 2005). Ayres' work has significantly influenced the development of the SMP, but the SMP must not be confused with Ayres Sensory Integration® (ASI®) because it does not meet all of the criteria of ASI fidelity (Parham *et al.* 2011).

This publication provides a primary focus on the area of sensory modulation, often referred to as the regulatory component of sensory integration and processing. The term sensory integration and processing (SIP) will be used as the term Ayres referred to as sensory integration, and what other leaders in the field of occupational therapy refer to as sensory processing, since these terms are used interchangeably. The SMP will be explored as a framework for conceptualizing and organizing interventions that may be helpful when working with people with dementia, as well as other populations when modified appropriately.

The changes that occur in the brain due to dementia are neurodegenerative. These changes negatively influence sensory integration and processing. When neurodegenerative changes occur, it is particularly important to consider ways in which to offer sensory-rich opportunities that are enjoyable to the person. Fostering these opportunities will support neurogenesis (growth or strengthening of the connections between neurons), feelings of safety and comfort, function, and participation.

Some people are able to remain healthy and vibrant throughout much of older adulthood. While this publication focuses primarily on use of the SMP with people with dementia, the SMP is also used with adolescents and adults of all ages and ability levels. Thus, many of the concepts and strategies contained within this book may be helpful to a wide variety of individuals across the lifespan. Adaptations to the SMP must be made to address individual preferences, age, and medical, cultural, religious, contextual, and environmental considerations.

Sensory deprivation

Due to the neurodegenerative changes that occur when a person experiences dementia, and other potentially co-existing conditions, there is frequently a decline in the ability to receive and efficiently process sensory input. Even when a person's brain is healthy, when human beings do not receive the amount and type of sensory input they require daily, degeneration and deconditioning may occur. People with neurodegenerative diseases, such as dementia, must be given opportunities for active engagement in sensory-rich activities and experiences that they find pleasant. The inability to obtain the amount and type of sensory input one needs, to the degree that it causes harm to the nervous system, is sometimes referred to as sensory deprivation. When sensory deprivation takes place, problems with cognition (e.g., confusion, hallucinations, delusions), emotion regulation, sensory processing and integration (e.g., coordination, balance [equilibrium]), motor performance, sensitivities, aggression, self-injury, and other difficult conditions and behaviors may emerge. Typically, the longer sensory deprivation occurs, the worse the corresponding symptoms and behaviors will become. Therefore, it is important to assess for possible signs of sensory deprivation, since it often goes unnoticed. Sensory supportive care, experiential opportunities throughout the daily routine, and sensory supportive physical environments are used to help decrease the possibility of sensory deprivation (Wood, Womack, & Hooper 2009).

The sensory processing umbrella

According to Miller *et al.* (2001), sensory processing is an umbrella term used to describe the following overarching categories of sensory processing:

- Sensory modulation

- Sensory discrimination

- Sensory-based motor performance

Sensory modulation

Sensory modulation is a neurophysiological process directly related to the ability to self-regulate. Therefore, it is commonly referred to as the *regulatory component* of sensory processing. The nervous system's ability to regulate and organize sensations supports the ability to make adaptive and graded responses without over- or under-responding. Sensory modulation also supports the ability to pay attention to "relevant" stimuli, while shutting out "irrelevant" stimuli, and it supports the ability to function within an "optimal" range of arousal.

According to Miller *et al.* (*ibid.*, p. 57), sensory modulation is the capacity to regulate and organize the degree, intensity, and nature of responses to sensory input in a graded and adaptive manner. This allows the individual to achieve and maintain an optimal range of performance and to adapt to challenges in daily life.

Each of the sensory systems receives and responds to stimulation in a manner that is unique to each individual and corresponds to the state of their nervous system at any point in time.

Dr. Winnie Dunn (2001) created a four-quadrant model demonstrating the different ways in which sensory modulation may be categorized. Within this quadrant model there is both a neurological and a behavioral response continuum. The four quadrant areas are:

- *Sensory sensitivity* and *sensation avoiding*: indicative of having a low neurological threshold for stimulation (easily notices or is bothered by stimulation)

- *Low registration* and *sensory seeking*: indicative of having a high neurological threshold for stimulation (difficulty perceiving and being aware of stimulation)

The ability to identify a person's specific patterns of sensory integration and processing requires assessment by a professional skilled in this area (e.g., occupational therapist, physical therapist).

Sensory sensitivity

Sensory sensitivity refer to when a person is more sensitive to a given stimulus than others in their age range, and may occur in one or multiple sensory systems. When a sensory sensitivity is specific to a particular sensory system, its effect is isolated to that area; for example, being sensitive to sounds (auditory system), certain tastes or smells (gustatory and olfactory systems), temperatures, or the feeling of being touched (tactile system). It is also possible to be hyper-sensitive across multiple systems, such as someone who is bothered by touch (tactile system), loud noises (auditory system), and bright lights (visual system). People with dementia may become easily overwhelmed by certain types of stimulation or when exposed to a lot of stimulation for a prolonged period of time. Some examples of various types of stimulation that people with dementia are often hyper-sensitive to include: visual stimulation (lighting, chaos in the environment), movement (transfers, walking, being moved), certain scents, loud noises, feeling too cold or too hot, and being touched or washed during self-care routines. When caregivers are aware of a client's specific hyper-sensitivities, they can help minimize the person's exposure to bothersome experiences, and be more deliberate about strategies that might help a person tolerate bothersome stimuli when necessary (e.g., during self-care tasks, to increase social and leisure participation).

Sensation avoiding

When people with dementia are bothered by stimulation of any kind, they may try to avoid situations or experiences. While a person is avoiding sensation they may refuse, curse, cry, scream, try to leave the situation, or even strike out in an attempt to stop what they perceive to be a negative experience. Understanding what part of the experience is bothersome can provide valuable information that caregivers can use to brainstorm creative ways in which to either help the person tolerate the stimulation or to minimize the degree of stimulation that is bothersome so that the person can remain as present and comfortable as possible.

Low registration

Low registration is a type of sensory modulation (regulatory) pattern whereby a person requires more stimulation than someone their age, similar to sensation seeking, but instead they do not necessarily seek out that stimulation. They may seem aloof, daydream a lot, and appear to lack the motivation or initiative to engage in activities that will give them the stimulation necessary to feel more regulated. Those who have low registration do not notice stimulation as much as others and it can be difficult for them to pay attention or concentrate during different activities. Similar to the other sensory modulation types, low registration may occur in one sensory system or multiple systems. It can be arduous to discern whether low registration is a modulation issue or if the behaviors observed are actually due to a problem with sensory discrimination.

Sensory seeking

Sensory seeking is evident when a person needs more stimulation of a certain type or types than people of the same age range. Sensory seeking may be part of the picture when a person is demonstrating self-stimulatory behaviors, refuses to stop using or doing something, or is in need of a particular type of stimulation due to not receiving enough in their daily routine (sensory deprivation, deconditioning).

Levels of severity

Difficulties with sensory processing are further categorized by levels of severity: mild, moderate, or severe. When sensory processing symptoms are mild, there is minimal impact on the person's ability to function. When the symptoms are more moderate, there is typically a negative effect on function and participation in roles and daily activities. Severe symptoms of sensory processing impact most areas of the person's life, including feelings of safety, wellness, and participation. In addition, when someone is not feeling well, is stressed, or is upset, symptom severity tends to increase (e.g., mild sensitivity turns into a more severe sensitivity in response to stress). People of all ages can relate to feeling ill and wanting to lower the lights, move to a quiet and less chaotic environment, and rest. For those whose daily life experiences are already overwhelming, not feeling well or being emotionally upset can significantly compound sensory integration and processing patterns. Feeling overwhelmed by any number of sensory-related triggers is particularly difficult for a person with dementia due to the combined challenge presented by sensory and cognitive problems, and potentially others too (e.g., physical challenges).

Sensory discrimination

Sensory discrimination refers to the ability to distinguish between distinct types of stimuli, across each of the different sensory systems. Sensory discrimination is not the same as sensory acuity because it occurs beyond the receptor level, at the level of the brain. For instance, the ability to tell whether something is soft, rough, light, heavy, hot, cold, sour, sweet, bright, dark, painful, noxious, or comforting depends not only on the receptors efficiently receiving the information but also on the ability to take the information obtained at the receptor level to the brain, where the salient qualities and gradations of the stimuli is processed further. It is the information received by the sensory receptors of each of the sensory systems that goes beyond the receptor level to be processed further (discrimination), and is then sent to the higher levels of the brain (cortical level) where we become more aware of multisensory perceptions (perception).

Gravitational insecurity

One type of sensory processing pattern that is commonly seen with many people with dementia is referred to as gravitational insecurity, which is primarily related to the functioning of the vestibular system. As discussed on page 32, the vestibular system is your own personal GPS, and is primarily responsible for balance, equilibrium, and spatial awareness (among other things). See the earlier section, "Vestibular system: sense of space, balance, and movement," for more information on its functions. Gravitational insecurity continues to be explored as a concept and the literature to date presents two different possible causes for it. One possible cause is when the person is hyper-sensitive to movement due to hyper-sensitivity in the vestibular system. When a person's vestibular system is hyper-sensitive it means that movement can feel overwhelming and there is often an increased fear of falling. When a person is hyper-sensitive to movement, feelings of fear frequently arise when they are moved. Imagine walking along a balance beam, but having difficulty with balance, confusion, vision, and spatial awareness, and having someone come along to move you in any way. Many people with dementia may become defensive when moved for this reason, and can strike out at caregivers when they are trying to help them change position, or perform transfers, self-care routines, stretching activities, and ambulation.

Providing caregivers with information about gravitational insecurity helps them understand why they are seeing certain behaviors. This knowledge will help them create strategies to ensure that a person feels safe and supported during movement activities and, consequently, that person will be less apt to demonstrate fearful responses (screaming, hitting, kicking).

Another potential cause of gravitational insecurity is having problems with sensory discrimination. When a person is struggling to discriminate between the types of stimuli experienced, the world can be a confusing and scary place to navigate. Therefore, having difficulty with vestibular discrimination impacts the ability to feel safe during activities or caregiving interventions requiring movement. The vestibular system is also interconnected with other sensory systems that play a role in the ability to feel safe when moving or being moved. Thus, it is essential to work with rehabilitation professionals to identify the type of difficulty the client is experiencing when they appear to have gravitational insecurity or demonstrate fearful or aggressive behaviors during any type of movement.

Sensory-based motor performance

Sensory-based motor performance refers to how the proprioceptive, tactile, vestibular, and visual systems support motor performance, thereby working together to help us move our bodies efficiently, safely, and functionally. When a person has issues with sensory discrimination, in any of the sensory systems that primarily support movement, they will negatively impact sensory-based motor performance. These systems work together to support the following:

- Body coordination
- Muscle tone
- Body positioning
- Balance and equilibrium
- Spatial awareness
- Directionality
- Body awareness
- Muscle strength
- Praxis

As the symptoms of dementia progress and increase in severity, a person's sensory-motor abilities are impacted. Our movement senses help us safely move our bodies, feel balanced, and perform efficient movements (navigate the stairs, perform activities requiring fine motor movements, anticipate the need for movement). People with dementia frequently experience changes in one or more of the sensory systems due to problems with acuity and/ or brain damage resulting from stroke or other types of insult or injury. Changes in function and behavior will depend largely on the areas of the brain impacted and the severity of that impact. It is common to observe difficulty with coordination, balance, spatial awareness, and the ability to communicate effectively as dementia progresses.

Praxis refers to the ability to sequence our actions through the steps necessary to complete any given activity, and is directly correlated with sensory-motor skills and the ability to discriminate sensory stimulation effectively. It is typical to see difficulty with praxis skills as dementia progresses to the moderate and severe stages. The coordination and sequencing of motor actions are required to eat and swallow without choking, walk safely, follow the steps required to complete a craft activity, and carry out self-care tasks (dressing, eating, bathing, grooming)—and rely (in part) on sensory-motor skills.

Assessment by a rehabilitation professional can aid in the determination of which sensory and motor systems are impacted so that rehabilitation services, daily activities, and compensatory strategies can be identified to help the person maintain skills for as long as possible and to ensure safety, participation, and quality of life as dementia progresses.

Evidence-based practice: sensory-based interventions

There is increasing evidence to support the use of sensory-based interventions with people with dementia. According to Padilla (2011), the skilled use of sensory approaches helps people with dementia make sense of their experiences and environments, which at times can be disorienting and confusing. In addition, sensory-based interventions have been found to encourage participation in activities of daily living (eating, bathing, dressing) by helping clients to feel more calm and relaxed, and less agitated (*ibid.*). King (2012) demonstrated that sensory-based interventions can decrease agitation and support active task participation. Several other researchers have shown that short-term, positive behavior changes, and increased social interaction and participation, are evident when using sensory-based approaches (Calkins 2005; Chen *et al.* 2013; Doble & Vania 2009; Dowling *et al.* 1997; Hope 1997; Hope & Waterman 1998; Klages *et al.* 2011; Locke & Mudford 2010; Sánchez *et al.* 2013; Staal *et al.* 2007).

Aman and Thomas (2009) revealed that a three-week exercise program, conducted three times per week in a nursing home setting, decreased agitation scores and improved six-meter walk times with people with severe cognitive impairment. The exercise program consisted of 30 minutes of exercise per session (5 minutes of aerobic exercises and 15 minutes of resistance exercises). It is interesting that many studies demonstrating the positive results of exercise do not mention the sensory systems involved, yet it is clear that while exercising the proprioceptive, vestibular, tactile, and visual systems are highly engaged. Knowing the different types of sensory input that support specific activities and outcomes is important in identifying other types of activity that provide similar input in order to expand upon the strategies that may be helpful.

In another study, by Cohen-Mansfield, Libin, and Marx (2007), non-pharmacological interventions were specifically designed to fulfill a need that matched the client's cognitive, sensory, and physical abilities, and lifelong habits and roles. The implementation of these individualized interventions resulted in decreased agitation and increased pleasure and interest in the chosen activities. Livingston *et al.* (2014) conducted a systematic review of 160 research studies that all focused on reducing agitation in dementia care. The literature review revealed that person-centered care, communication skills, sensory-based therapeutic activities, and dementia care mapping helped to reduce agitation in people with dementia living in care homes.

In summary, there is a growing body of research that supports the positive effect of sensory-based interventions on mood and the ability to engage in activities of daily living, leisure, and social experiences, and their reduction of agitation in people with dementia. The SMP provides a framework for the implementation of sensory-based approaches with people with dementia.

Chapter 3

The Sensory Modulation Program

The Sensory Modulation Program (SMP) is a framework that provides a general methodology for integrating the use of sensory modulation-related interventions with different populations. This chapter provides an overview of the SMP components and the subsequent chapters outline each in more detail. The SMP was initially developed for use with adolescents, adults, and older persons. The author has adapted it for use with people of all ages, including those with dementia, and for application across a wide variety of settings, such as inpatient, long-term care, skilled nursing, forensic, school, and home settings (Champagne 2011). The SMP has also been adapted and used as part of palliative care services, to support pain management, and with clients at the end stage of life, as an adjunct to other interventions. Describing and explaining the benefits of using the SMP with people with dementia is the purpose of this book.

With the onset of dementia, changes in sensory perception and cognitive ability make it increasingly difficult to make sense of everyday life experiences. As dementia progresses, clients and caregivers increasingly rely on professional support and strategies that assist the person with dementia to feel more safe and supported and able to function. The SMP provides a roadmap for how to implement individualized sensory-based approaches that support a variety of goals: feeling safe and secure, increasing self-coherence and self-regulation, identifying and implementing cognitive and sensory-based supports, and increasing the ability to engage in meaningful roles, routines, activities, and relationships to the best of the person's ability (*ibid.*). Additionally, the skilled, responsible, and client-centered use of the SMP supports the development of a strong therapeutic relationship between the client, caregiver(s), and involved staff, given that the therapeutic use of self is the most important SMP component. The therapeutic use of self is a term referring to how a caregiver or member of staff uses an empathic approach and aspects of body language to support the client (e.g., energy level, body position, tone of voice).

When using the SMP, obtaining supplemental training or consultation to adapt and apply its concepts and techniques may be necessary. Although several of the interventions appear easy to incorporate into the care provided, understanding the potential safety considerations and contra-indications when using many of the different sensory-based approaches and when modifying and enhancing physical environments is critical. Whenever possible, working collaboratively with rehabilitation professionals (e.g., occupational or physical therapists) trained in the area of sensory integration and processing is recommended to help ensure the safe and skilled implementation of the SMP.

Components of the Sensory Modulation Program

The SMP is comprised of seven components and can be used with individuals and for programmatic application (Champagne 2011). The main components of the SMP are:

- Therapeutic use of self

- Sensory-based assessments, as part of the overall assessment process (to support sensory-based goal setting and intervention planning)

- Sensorimotor activities

- Sensory-based modalities

- Sensory diet (sensory strategies strategically integrated into the daily routine)

- Environmental modifications and enhancements

- Client and caregiver involvement and education

Many healthcare professionals implement one or more of the SMP components without necessarily implementing the program in its entirety, which can prove to be helpful at times. This may occur when a client is introduced to a specific sensory modality (weighted doll, pet therapy), sensorimotor activity (stretching, cooking or craft activity), or sensory room without necessarily having the SMP used in a more comprehensive manner. Complementary or integrative therapies are also sensory-based and considered part of the SMP. The skilled and individualized application of the entirety of the SMP, however, is recommended for optimal results. As an introduction to the SMP, an overview of each of the different components is provided, and the following chapters provide more detail and corresponding resources.

Therapeutic use of self

The therapeutic use of self refers to the intentional way in which a person approaches and interacts with another to foster trust and develop a relationship over time. The therapeutic use of self is often used by caregiver(s), staff, and other types of care provider. Whether the person providing care is a loved one or a healthcare professional, the therapeutic use of self is foundational to providing compassionate, kind, and holistic care. The therapeutic use of self requires the use of one's energy, body positioning, and whole being in a respectful, empathetic, and deeply caring way in order to benefit the client and caregiver(s), and it is the most important component of the SMP (Champagne 2011; Yamaguchi, Maki, & Tamagami 2010). The therapeutic relationship begins by establishing a rapport and an alliance with the client and any involved caregiver(s). The therapeutic relationship is central to the ability to help the client and caregiver(s) to feel safe and supported, particularly as the client's needs progress.

People with dementia become increasingly vulnerable as the disease progresses, so it is critical that a trusting relationship is established and maintained over time—a strong therapeutic alliance is at the heart of client-centered care (Geller & Porges 2014). To be client-centered requires focusing on the person and their loved ones in a way that makes the therapeutic relationship, client's privacy, individualized needs and goals, preferences, beliefs, values, dignity, and respect *central* to the caregiving process. In this way, the client's wishes and needs are predominant, rather than the primary focus being on dementia or some other variable, such as the practitioner's preferences, values, or biases (Veselinova 2014). Using a client-centered approach as part of the strong emphasis on the therapeutic use of self requires that the client must not only have their basic needs met, but should also feel that they are deeply cared for, respected, and central to caregiving decision making and care received.

Attunement is at the heart of a client-centered, relational, trauma-informed approach (for more information on trauma-informed care, refer to Chapter 1). Attunement is the ability to create a connected relationship with a person at any age and ability level. Attunement is commonly used in the attachment literature when referring to how the mother–infant relationship is established and evolves over time. To attune to a person with dementia is also important because, first and foremost, the client is a person who needs connection, compassion, reassurance, and comfort. In order to create an attuned relationship, intentionality in the way that verbal and nonverbal communication skills are used is key. Treating older adults with respect, and in an age and culturally appropriate manner, is essential to fostering effective and respectful communication, which is foundational to attunement. The following list provides examples of some of the components of verbal communication that must be considered when working with people with dementia (McEvoy & Plant 2014):

- Choosing appropriate language

- Moderating tone of voice

- Moderating volume of voice

- Speaking clearly

- Slowing speed/rate of speech

- Explaining or discussing one concept or step at a time

- Asking short, direct questions

- Considering whether open- or closed-ended questions are most appropriate as dementia progresses

- Using music and singing

- Being aware of and showing respect for cultural and religious issues

- Considering the age appropriateness of all interactions

While many people recognize the therapeutic effects of music for people with dementia, the use of singing is another verbal communication strategy (Chatterton, Baker, & Morgan, 2010; Hammar *et al.* 2010, 2011).

Across the lifespan, most communication is actually conducted non-verbally. Some of the nonverbal communication components to pay attention to when interacting with people with dementia are:

- Active, empathic, and compassionate listening (show you are interested, attentive, sincere)

- Pleasant demeanor

- Positive attitude towards client and others

- Open and relaxed energy and body language

- Eye contact (caring, direct, interested, sincere)

- Caring forms of touch

- A slower pace

- Gestures (clear, caring, and directive)

- Head nods

- Attention to body positioning and posture (position self within the person's visual field, approach from the front)

As dementia progresses, it becomes increasingly necessary to focus one's attention on the nonverbal communication of the client, in addition to what they are able to communicate verbally (e.g., changes in emotions, likes/dislikes, degree of functionality under certain conditions, identification of what helps). It is also important to give the client ample time to process information and to respond. Modifying one's approach to communicating and observing how the person responds in different situations is strongly recommended. It becomes increasingly difficult for people with dementia to process information and communicate due to the changes that occur in the parts of the brain supporting these abilities (Jootun & McGhee 2011; McEvoy & Plant 2014; de Vries 2013). Supporting the therapeutic relationship through ongoing attention to the use of self, which includes modifications to communicating with and understanding the experiences of people with dementia as the disease progresses, is central to the successful implementation of the SMP.

Sensory-based assessments

Sensory-based assessments are used to help obtain the information needed to determine a person's unique sensory processing patterns, which inform the ability to create an individualized SMP. Assessment also helps to identify safety and medical concerns that need to be taken into account for each individual before using sensory-based strategies (e.g., allergies, fragile skin, respiratory problems). Assessment information is collected to help identify the person's specific needs, strengths, and goals. Assessment information supports the reasoning and decision-making process regarding why particular sensory-based strategies might be considered potentially helpful or not. For instance, if a person is bothered by tactile forms of input that would be important to know prior to initiating the use of sensory-based strategies offering those types of stimulation. Once the assessment information is obtained, a variety of sensorimotor activities, sensory-based modalities, and environmental supports are explored that are believed to be potentially helpful. For some individuals, offering different sensory strategies requires slow initiation, one at a time and over a period of time, to ensure they are not overwhelmed. Introducing one strategy at a time also allows for the identification of those that are more or less helpful. As sensory strategies are identified as aiding the individual (or not), this information is tracked and helpful strategies are compiled into an individualized daily routine, a *sensory diet*. The sensory diet is updated over time as the person's likes, dislikes, needs, and goals continue to be identified and/or change. For more information on assessment, refer to Chapter 4.

Sensorimotor activities

Sensorimotor activities include a wide range of activities that provide increased opportunity for sensory and motor stimulation, specific to the individual's needs and goals. There are endless possibilities because everything we experience is sensory-based in one way or another, and most activities require some sort of movement component as well. When using vision, your eyes require the eye musculature to help scan and focus vision, the ears contain tiny muscles that support hearing, and even breathing requires muscles to support respiration! Meaningful activities that foster artistic and creative expression, as well as movement-based activities, are examples of sensorimotor activities often used with people with dementia (Cowl & Gaugler 2014; Pitkälä *et al.* 2013; Pöllänen & Hirsimäki 2014). What makes a sensorimotor activity part of the SMP, rather than a mere diversionary activity, is that there is a skilled and strategic rationale for how it will help the individual meet their therapeutic goals. Below are a few examples of sensorimotor activities:

- Doing art activities
- Doing crafts

- Listening to music

- Playing an instrument

- Exercise and stretch activities

- Playing target games (bowling, ring toss)

- Playing bingo or card games

- Dancing (seated or standing)

- Planning or participating in social events or parties

- Petting an animal (dog or cat)

- Weaving, sorting, or folding activities

- Undertaking self-care activities

Again, the sensorimotor activities offered as part of the SMP must be those that are sensory supportive, meaningful, purposeful, age appropriate for the person(s) involved, and specific to the client's needs, values, and goals (Letts *et al.* 2011). Simply because someone has dementia does not mean that random, purposeless activities that have no meaning are appropriate. It is certainly possible to engage people with dementia in meaningful and purposeful activities (e.g., helping to polish silverware, fold napkins for mealtimes, sort laundry, help set up for activities or meals).

Spiritual and cultural issues must also be taken into consideration when planning for and offering care to people with dementia, including sensorimotor activities. Spiritually-based activities are used to help clients remain engaged in rituals and activities that have been deeply meaningful to them, such as visits from clergy, attending places of worship or watching services on television, religious holiday observance and participation in associated events, and access to items specific to their faith (the Bible, Quran, Torah, rosary beads, gospel music, and so on). Awareness of the cultural norms and values of the client and their family provides a greater understanding of their beliefs related to dementia, views on accepting help/care, and patterns of communication, and supports the ability to offer culturally sensitive activities such as cooking preferred foods, organizing holiday celebrations, offering preferred music selections, and more!

Sensory-based modalities

A modality is a tool, object, or piece of equipment used for a specific therapeutic purpose. Sensory-based modalities, like other parts of the SMP, aim to help individuals self-organize and meet specific needs and goals (Champagne 2011). Sensory modalities that may be used with people with dementia include:

- Clinical aromatherapy
- Expressive art therapies (music, art, movement)
- Light therapy
- Pet therapy
- Weighted modalities (weighted blanket, lap pad, shawl, or vest)
- Brushing or bean bag-tapping techniques
- Biofeedback

A growing body of evidence reveals the effectiveness of some of the more common types of sensory-based modality. Sensory-based modalities that have been researched with geriatric populations, including people with dementia, and found to be effective include clinical aromatherapy, music therapy, pet therapy (Perkins *et al*. 2008; Williams & Jenkins 2008), and light therapy (Dowling *et al*. 2007). In research articles, sensory-based modalities are also referred to as types of complementary, integrative, or non-pharmacological intervention. More research is needed to demonstrate the broad range of sensory-based modalities that are helpful to people with dementia, including corresponding safety considerations and contra-indications.

For safety reasons, additional training is often required before using therapeutic sensory-based modalities. Additionally, in medical or skilled nursing facilities, policies and procedures for the use of sensory-based modalities may be required. Medical and clinical safety recommendations and contra-indications must be identified and taken into consideration before using sensory-based modalities with people with dementia and other medical or mental health conditions. Working with medical and rehabilitation professionals can provide the expertise necessary to safely implement the use of sensory-based activities and modalities and to create policies and procedures for use.

Sensory diet

A sensory diet is a strategically planned routine that incorporates sensory-based strategies that promote feelings of safety, comfort, and calm, and support active participation in roles, routines, and activities (Wilbarger 1995). The term sensory diet is not meant to be restrictive, but rather refers to the range or menu of possible options that are helpful to the individual for a variety of therapeutic reasons (e.g., prevention, crisis de-escalation, to prepare and support the ability to engage in activities [preparatory], to maintain skills). A sensory diet refers to the strategic use of specific, sensory-based strategies throughout the daily routine to help meet the client's needs and goals. The following mini-case example demonstrates how a client's early morning routine and sensory-based interventions are woven into an individualized sensory diet as part of her plan of care.

Sandy's early morning routine: relevant assessment information

Sandy has tactile and oral sensitivities, and visual impairment, and requires a wheelchair for mobility. Sandy's husband reports that she has always been a "morning person," that breakfast is her favorite meal of the day, and that she wakes up at approximately 7:00 a.m. most days.

At approximately 7:00 a.m.:

- Once Sandy awakens, use a gentle yet cheerful tone of voice to greet her, "Good morning, Sandy," and provide an orientation to the day of the week, "It is Monday morning."

- Introduce yourself and what activity is coming next: "It is (your name) and I am here to help you get ready for breakfast."

- Ask her if she is ready to get up: "Would you like to get up and get ready for breakfast?"

- Give her time to feel fully awake and ready to sit up.

- Ask her: "Are you ready to sit up?" and if she is, slowly raise the head of her bed to the seated position after informing her that you will be doing so.

- Offer her a warm washcloth so that she can wipe her face.

- Provide her eye glasses so that she can see who is helping her, what is happening, and where things are located (to help her feel more oriented).

- Ask if she is ready to move to her wheelchair. If not, ask her what she would like to do first, offering two choices. If she is ready, move on to the next step.

- When she is ready to transfer to the wheelchair:

  - Approach Sandy from the front and, if more than one person is needed to help, introduce them and ensure they are also located within Sandy's visual field.
  - Approach her using caring mannerisms and at a relatively slow pace.
  - Provide a pre-warmed sheet and gently help her position it across her shoulders. Give her the ends of the sheet to hold on to so that she feels more secure. The use of the sheet will also decrease the possibility of a negative response to the many touches to her skin that may occur during a two-person transfer.
  - Gently carry out the two-person transfer to the wheelchair on a 1–3 count and provide ongoing reassurance as needed to ensure Sandy feels safe and secure.

This example demonstrates the first part of Sandy's sensory diet and highlights the significance of the therapeutic use of self and sensory-based strategies. Sandy's early morning routine is most successful when her caregivers are informed about and trained to provide her sensory diet in a skilled manner. While some may argue that such an approach takes too much time to implement, should Sandy become overwhelmed during her morning routine she may require an even greater level of support, and this may also negatively impact her quality of life.

The most intensive need for sensory-based support tends to be before and during transition times of the day (e.g., waking up/morning routines, changes of shift in care settings, getting ready for bed/going to sleep), when engaging in activities of daily living (e.g., bathing, dressing, toileting), and when trying to support leisure and social participation. In addition, when working with people with dementia, those who experience sundowning or gravitational insecurity (see below) often require additional support to maintain safety and decrease the potential for increased fearfulness, anxiety, paranoia, and aggressive behaviors.

Sundowning

People in the moderate to late stages of dementia experience a period in the day known as "sundowning," which typically occurs in the early to mid-afternoon. When a person experiences sundowning, they commonly feel more agitated, anxious, fearful, and paranoid. Sensory-based and other supportive strategies are frequently used before and during these times of day to help ease the related symptoms and corresponding behaviors. The goal of the SMP with people experiencing sundowning is to help them feel safe, secure, and comforted. Examples of sensory-based strategies for people experiencing sundowning include: sing-a-longs, walks, time in a sensory room, a weighted doll or stuffed animal, aromatherapy, snacks, and positive forms of distraction from fears and worries (Forbes & Gresham 2011). Visits from family members may also decrease the amount of distress.

Gravitational insecurity

Gravitational insecurity (GI) is a type of hyper-sensitivity to movement coupled with a defensive response that may be mild, moderate, or severe. It is important that caregivers of people with GI are educated on the subject, and that the client's sensory diet includes instructions for all involved caregivers. The instructions should describe the best way to engender feelings of safety and security whenever the individual is being moved, participating in transfers, engaging in activities that involve the feet leaving the ground, or being touched (self-care, ambulation, leisure). For more information on gravitational insecurity, refer to Chapter 2.

Environmental modifications and enhancements

The physical environment can be modified or enhanced in several ways to support people with dementia. Adaptive equipment, home modifications, enhancements to lighting, sound dampening acoustic panels, the addition of a large fish tank, and the creation and use of sensory rooms and carts are all examples of ways in which the environment can be used to support the sensory needs of people with dementia. Clients and caregivers can collaborate to identify creative approaches and organize spaces according to the client's needs and goals. Natural environments provide an additional means for offering sensory-supportive spaces, such as sensory gardens, outdoor exercise equipment, outdoor gliders, and more! Chapter 7 provides an in-depth review of information about environmental modifications and enhancements for use with people with dementia.

Client and caregiver involvement and education

The care provided to any population must be centered on the needs and goals of individuals and their caregiver(s). In order to meet this goal, clients and caregivers have to be included in any/all assessment processes, care planning, and care delivery. As dementia progresses, involved caregivers often increase the level of support they offer because the client becomes more vulnerable and dependent on others. Having involved caregivers and people who know the client really well (and who are authorized to participate) is extremely valuable to both the client and all involved in their care. Caregivers are critical to maintaining quality of life and decreasing the probability of depression, agitation, and aggression over time. Staff can support the client and caregiver by providing education as needed, and in aiding the understanding of loved ones regarding what to expect as the disease progresses.

People with dementia and their caregivers rely on the education professionals provide. Educational materials about the types and stages of dementia, various kinds of interventions and supports that may be useful at the different stages, medical issues that may arise, prevention and maintenance techniques, and other caregiver supports are examples of information sought out by caregivers. Additionally, when using a sensory-based approach and the SMP, information about changes in sensory perception and how sensory-based strategies can be helpful to people with dementia is also necessary. For those providing care to their loved ones at home, it is essential to provide a sensory diet and home program, together with examples of the rationale for their use as provided in the research literature; recommendations for home modifications and sensory-based enhancements; and information about safety considerations.

Caregivers may also need support and resources for themselves; for this reason, a wealth of information is provided in the Resources section at the end of the book.

Sensory Modulation Program goals

The goals of the SMP are broad-based in order to be easily adapted and used with a wide variety of populations. Accordingly, the SMP goals provided in this chapter have been modified for working with people with dementia.

Goal 1. Facilitating self-awareness: identification of sensory-based patterns and goals.

- A qualified individual completes a comprehensive assessment in collaboration with the client and involved caregiver, and includes identification of the client's sensory-based patterns and preferences in addition to other areas of assessment (strengths, interests, values, medical concerns, cognitive ability, trauma history, etc.). Whenever possible, the assessment process includes:

    - Chart review
    - Interview of the client to the extent that that is possible

- Information from the guardian or other individuals that the guardian has given permission to use
- Observation of the ability to participate in roles, routines, and activities
- Assessment of the impact of the client's sensory processing patterns and preferences on relational capacities, attention span/orientation, mood, safety, comfort, and behavior
- Any other assessments appropriate to the client's ability level and areas of need (e.g., balance, fall risk)
- Interpretation of the assessment results and recommendations for potential areas of need/concern, goals, and interventions

Goal 2. Sensory strategizing: exploring, planning, and implementing.

- Assist the individual in exploring sensory-based strategies that may help foster self-organization, ensure safety, and support the person's specific needs and goals

- Identify initial sensory-based strategies to try as part of a sensory diet (throughout the daily routine), and also those to be used for crisis de-escalation purposes (as needed)

- Collaboratively create and implement the initial sensory diet (with client and involved caregivers), incorporating sensory-based strategies identified as helpful

- Provide all caregivers with the client's initial sensory diet (a strategic routine that is comprised of sensory-based prevention, preparatory, and crisis de-escalation strategies) including an emphasis on the individual's strengths, interests, activities, needs, and goals; provide the training and communication tools necessary to support the skillful implementation of the initial sensory diet by involved staff and caregivers

- Monitor the effectiveness of the initial sensory diet, based on the client's responsivity to the sensory approaches being implemented, and update as needed

- Identify environmental modifications and enhancements

Goal 3. Skilled implementation of the SMP.

- Demonstrate active use of the SMP, individualized to support self-organization, safety, participation (roles, routines, activities), and quality of life, on the part of the individual, caregivers, and staff

- Assist the client and caregiver(s) in the skillful use of the SMP to help decrease unsafe behaviors (falls, agitation, aggression, self-injury)

Goal 4. Repertoire expansion: SMP modification.

- Re-assess and modify the SMP as the person's needs, preferences, and goals change over time (e.g., sensory diet, sensorimotor activities, sensory-based modalities, environmental modifications and enhancements, caregiver education and support)

Individual and programmatic applications of the Sensory Modulation Program

The SMP may be implemented individually and programmatically. As we have reviewed in this chapter so far, an individualized approach requires that each component of the SMP be implemented in an individualized manner, based on the client's assessment results, skilled observations, and ongoing interactions with the client and caregiver(s) to ensure effectiveness. After the initial assessment process is complete, exploration of sensorimotor activities and sensory-based modalities that correspond to each individual's needs and preferences helps to determine introductory sensory-based strategies. Over time, as strategies supportive of the client's preferences and goals are identified, those interventions are woven into the client's daily routine. Thus, preferred sensorimotor activities and sensory-based modalities, as well as strategies supporting activities of daily living, are worked into the client's sensory diet. Environmental enhancements, supports, and modifications that are, or may be, helpful to the individual are also instituted. As time progresses, the options utilized are reviewed and enhanced based on the client's response and staff and caregiver reports. Even when a client is unable to communicate, it is important to use skilled observation to determine whether changes should be made to enhance their SMP.

The story of June provides another example illustrating the institution of the SMP. June is an 87-year-old wife, mother, grandmother, and great-grandmother. Before getting married and becoming a mother and home-maker in her twenties, June worked as a telephone operator. Throughout her life she was highly skilled at cooking, sewing, knitting, and crocheting. She is currently demonstrating the symptoms of moderate to late stage dementia, and has therefore entered a skilled nursing facility (SNF). Prior to admission to the SNF, June was living at home with her family and provided with nursing care. Initially, she was fearful and demonstrated increased confusion while settling into the new living environment of the

SNF. She often called out for her husband and repeatedly stated "I am done with school and ready to go home now" while pacing up and down the hallways. Table 3.1 provides some examples of the assessment process and shows how some of the early strategies used as part of June's individualized SMP were identified and developed.

Table 3.1 Sensory Modulation Program: individual application

Sensory Modulation Program components	Individual application example: June
Therapeutic use of self	• Spent time with June and her primary caregiver getting to know her, the things she enjoys and dislikes, and identifying her supports.
Assessment	• Completed a chart review, had her family complete a safety tool (which includes sensory and trauma-informed care-related questions), completed cognitive, sensorimotor and balance-related observations.
Sensory diet	• After working with June and her primary caregiver to learn about her history, preferences, and needs, created and implemented an individualized daily routine incorporating sensory strategies. The plan is to implement the routine and modify/enhance it over time. The initial goal of implementing the sensory diet is to support feelings of comfort and safety, and increase participation.
Sensorimotor activities	• Provided a range of sensorimotor activities in group and individual sessions identified as meaningful to June (crafts, sorting fabrics/sewing supplies, sing-a-longs, walks outdoors in the garden).
Sensory modalities	• Staff worked with June and family members to identify the different modalities she liked: weighted doll, weighted wrap (shawl), aromatherapy (lavender), and dog therapy.
Environmental modifications and enhancements	• Adjusted the blinds/lighting and seating arrangement to minimize glare and loud or abrupt noises. • Ensured environmental supports and tools provide warmth at all times during activities of daily living (warm blankets, towels, and room temperature).
Client and caregiver involvement and education	• A family member helped to complete the safety tool and provided June's history, strengths, leisure and social interests, routine patterns and preferences, and previous traumatic stressors. A family member also assisted with introducing new activities and environmental supports with staff, to promote the therapeutic relationship and ensure that June feels safe and secure with staff. Caregiver education on the SMP and how it could be helpful to June was provided to family by staff.

To implement the SMP on a programmatic scale, a needs assessment is completed to identify how to integrate each of its aspects throughout the program's daily routine and to evaluate the physical environment. The programmatic schedule is reviewed to determine the client's needs and take in staff recommendations regarding whether what is being offered throughout the daily routine is fulfilling those needs, including the programming offered during transition times. Sensorimotor activities and sensory-based modalities that would be helpful for a broad range of clients are established. To ensure safe and skilled implementation, training is provided on the SMP, and policies and procedures are developed and enforced. Environmental modifications and enhancements are considered for the whole setting, including the possibility of creating a sensory room and sensory garden. The results of the needs assessment are used to institute the SMP on a programmatic scale. Training on how to implement the SMP with people with dementia, and in particular on how to incorporate a trauma-informed approach, is typically necessary. Table 3.2 outlines examples of ways in which to implement the SMP on a programmatic scale.

Table 3.2 Sensory Modulation Program implementation: programmatic application

Sensory Modulation Program components	Programmatic application example
Therapeutic use of self	• Provide education to staff on verbal, nonverbal, and sensory-based techniques that support the ability to create and maintain a therapeutic relationship with people with dementia and involved caregivers.
Assessment	• Conduct a needs assessment exploring all aspects of the program and areas that need to be addressed in order to skillfully implement the SMP programmatically (e.g., sensory and trauma-informed care-related assessments; sensory-based activity and equipment needs; documentation needs; necessary environmental renovations, modifications, and enhancements; staff training needs; policies and procedures required; referral sources for rehabilitation services).
Sensory diet	• Enhance the programmatic routine and offer sensory-based activities and supports during all transition times.
Sensorimotor activities	• Expand on the sensorimotor activities offered.
Sensory-based modalities	• Expand on the sensory-based modalities offered.
Environmental modifications and enhancements	• Enhance all areas of the physical environment to make them more sensory supportive (e.g., bedrooms, bathrooms, dining rooms, sensory rooms, sensory gardens).
Client and caregiver involvement and education	• Identify consistent ways in which to collaborate with the client and caregiver across all aspects of care delivery (assessment, goal setting, care planning and implementation, re-assessment over time).

In summary, using the SMP on both individual and programmatic scales allows for its comprehensive implementation and increases the probability of achieving the most favorable outcomes. It takes leadership commitment, strategic planning, funding, and time to institute the SMP on both individual and programmatic scales. When implementing the SMP in healthcare settings, collaborating with rehabilitation professionals (skilled in sensory integration and processing) can help the needs assessment process, offer staff training, pinpoint necessary equipment, assist in identifying essential environmental modifications and enhancements, and support the development of policies and procedures. Rehabilitation professionals can also provide the support and education needed to safely put the SMP into practice at home or in community-based settings.

Chapter 4

Assessment and Safety Considerations

If the doors of perceptions were cleansed, everything would appear as it is, infinite. ~ William Blake

Assessment is a process used to identify an individual's strengths, specific safety concerns, needs, care preferences, and goals. For people with dementia, the assessment process is typically conducted upon admission to a healthcare, rehabilitation, independent living, or nursing facility, and/or at the start of engagement with healthcare services in specific disciplines (social workers, doctors, nurses, rehabilitation professionals). The client and involved caregivers must be central to the assessment and care planning process. When creating an individualized sensory modulation program (SMP) with a client and involved caregiver(s), the assessment process is used to gather some of the following information:

- Meaningful life roles

- Personal strengths

- Medical and trauma histories

- Daily routine (general and specific information)

- Likes and dislikes

- Work, leisure, and social histories

- Cultural and spiritual considerations

- Assessment of cognitive ability

- Assessment of sensory-based patterns and tendencies

- Assessment of environmental needs and supports

Safety considerations and trauma history

While sensory-based interventions can be very helpful, people may have safety considerations that are critical to their health and overall well-being. The following list provides examples of common safety concerns that must be taken into consideration before initiating the use of sensory-based approaches with people with dementia (please note: this list is not all-inclusive):

- Stage of dementia (cognitive and communication ability levels)

- Allergies (medication, food, environmental)

- Fragile skin or wounds

- Type and degree of arthritis

- Fractures or broken bones

- Balance or gait problems

- Fall risk

- Cardiac, respiratory, and other medical conditions

- Swallow precautions

- Triggers related to past traumatic or other mental health experiences

- Seizure history

- Evidence of the effects of deconditioning or sensory deprivation that may have occurred

- Medications and potential side effects

A careful review of the client's medical records helps to ensure that caregivers are aware of all known and potential safety and medical concerns. Whenever there are any safety concerns, prior to the use of sensory-based approaches (including implementation of the SMP) it is important to determine whether it is necessary to obtain a doctor's order or to follow any special recommendations made by medical or rehabilitation professionals or other sources in advance (e.g., a weighted blanket may not be suitable for someone with fragile skin, weakness, or respiratory concerns). There may be different requirements for the use of certain sensory-based modalities in various states or countries as well (e.g., clinical aromatherapy, weighted modalities). Therefore, it is crucial to be informed and check with each organization's administration prior to use.

A person's trauma history and related triggers and warning signs should be assessed in order to provide care that is trauma sensitive. When working with people with trauma histories, it is helpful to use a safety tool (MacLaughlin & Stromberg 2012), also referred to in some settings as a de-escalation tool. The safety tool is a questionnaire used to gather information about a person's trauma history, triggers, warning signs, and any helpful strategies. In addition, safety tools ask questions that may serve as a form of advanced directive in regards to preferences in different situations, such as who to contact in the case of restraint use or medical emergency. Similar to administering other assessment or screening tools when working with people with dementia, it is advantageous to have people who know the client well help complete the safety tool. The information gained from the safety tool is used to provide more individualized care.

The Trauma Informed Safety Questionnaire (TISC) is one example of a safety tool used with clients with dementia or who have difficulty communicating. Whenever possible, the client participates in providing as much information as possible when completing the TISC. When a client is unable to complete the TISC, people who know the individual well are asked to provide as much information as possible (with the client's permission). The TISC is provided in Appendix A.

Sensory-based assessment and screening

Assessment tools are used to gather information to support the assessment process (e.g., questionnaires, checklists, vital signs or other medical monitoring tools). While few specific sensory-based assessment tools have been created for use with people with dementia, nevertheless some do exist. People who are in the early stages of dementia are often able to be active participants in the assessment process because they are able to communicate and answer questions accurately. Thus, during the early stages of dementia, caregivers may offer supplemental information, but the client is the person providing the majority of the information on their own behalf. Some of the sensory processing-related assessment tools that may be useful when working with people in the earlier stages of dementia are the self-questionnaires listed below:

- Adolescent/Adult Sensory Profile (Brown & Dunn 2002)

- Adult/Adolescent Sensory History (May-Benson 2014)

- Sensory Defensiveness Questionnaire (Champagne 2011)

- Sensory Modulation Tool (Champagne 2011)

- The Sensory Processing Caregiver Checklist: Adults and Older Persons (Champagne 2017)

As dementia progresses, it becomes increasingly difficult to interview or use self-questionnaires with the client as a result of the cognitive and communication challenges they face. As cognitive and communication abilities diminish, the self-rating questionnaires that are mentioned above are sometimes used with caregivers in order to see if any of the questions can be answered. When appropriate, it is possible to modify the assessment and screening tools in order to obtain the specific information needed from the client or caregiver(s). However, it is important to realize that, when standardized or evidence-based assessment tools are modified, they are no longer evidence-based assessment tools; instead they become tools that are used solely to gather or obtain information.

Although clients must be included in the assessment process whenever possible, over time increased reliance on skilled, clinical observations and caregiver reports are increasingly relied upon and become critical parts of the assessment process. The Sensory Processing Caregiver Checklist: Adults and Older Persons (SPCC) is a questionnaire created to be used with caregivers who know the client well; it is also used to help guide clinical observations as part of the assessment process. The SPCC is designed to help explore sensory modulation patterns (under- and over-responsivity patterns), sensory discrimination patterns, and self-stimulatory and self-injurious behaviors. The SPCC is provided in Appendix B.

Another example of a sensory processing-related caregiver questionnaire, created specifically for use with caregivers of people with dementia or other significant cognitive impairments, is the Caregiver Questionnaire (Champagne 2011). This tool asks a host of questions that the caregiver may or may not be able to answer. The goal of the Caregiver Questionnaire is to obtain as much information as caregivers (loved ones and involved staff) are able to provide to support the assessment process. Different categories of question explore the following issues:

- Sensory-based preferences (personal and environmental)

- Daily routine and self-care preferences

- Work and leisure history and preferences

- Cultural and spiritual history and preferences

- Trauma history

Last, but not least, another caregiver tool that collects information related to sensory processing is the Sensory Integration Inventory–Revised (SII-R; Reisman & Hanschu 1992). The SII-R was initially created for use with adults with developmental disabilities but is occasionally used with other adult populations experiencing cognitive or communication difficulties. It is used to help gather information about proprioceptive, tactile, and vestibular processing and related functional performance areas and self-injurious behaviors.

Balance and fall risk assessments

The following are additional examples of assessment and screening tools that may be used by rehabilitation professionals to help support the assessment process when working with older persons, including people with dementia.

Balance:

- Berg Balance Scale (www.strokecenter.org/wp-content/uploads/2011/08/berg.pdf)

- Tinetti Assessment Tool: Balance & Gait (http://ptclinic.com/websites/991/files/TinettiBalanceAndGaitAssessment.pdf)

- Elderly Mobility Scale

Fall risk:

- Johns Hopkins Home Health Care and Acute Care Tools (www.hopkinsmedicine.org/institute_nursing/models_tools/fall_risk.html)

- Home Fall Prevention Checklist (www.cdc.gov/HomeandRecreationalSafety/pubs/English/booklet_Eng_desktop-a.pdf)

Dementia, cognitive, and other assessments

Dementia, cognitive, and other types of assessment and screening tools are used with people with dementia to look at both cognitive ability and the various types of change that occur as time progresses. A variety of assessment tools used to assess and monitor concerns related to dementia are provided (please note: these lists are not all-inclusive).

Dementia screenings

Examples of common screening tools, specifically used to assess for the signs and stages of dementia include:

- Alzheimer's Disease Assessment Scale (Rosen, Mohs, & Davis 1984)

- Blessed Information-Memory-Concentration Test (www.strokecenter.org/wp-content/uploads/2011/08/bd_imct.pdf)

- Clinical Dementia Rating Scale (http://alzheimer.wustl.edu/adrc2/Images/CDRWorksheet.pdf)

- Dementia Severity Rating Scale (www.alz.org/careplanning/downloads/dsrs-scale.pdf)

- Mini-mental Screening Tool (Folstein, Folstein, & McHugh 1975)

Cognitive assessments: executive functioning

- Allen Cognitive Assessment Battery (Allen, Earhart, & Blue 1999)

- Cognitive Performance Test (Burns 2006)

- Lowenstein Occupational Therapy Cognitive Assessment—Geriatric Version (Katz, Averbuch, & Erez 2011)

Activities of daily living and safety scales

- Activities of Daily Living (ADL) (http://consultgeri.org/try-this/general-assessment/issue-2.pdf)

- Functional Activities Questionnaire: Older Adults with Dementia (www.alz.org/careplanning/downloads/functional-activities-questionnaire.pdf)

- Instrumental Activities of Daily Living (IADL) (http://consultgeri.org/try-this/dementia/issue-d13.pdf)

- Safety Assessment Checklist (www.alz.org/careplanning/downloads/safety-assess-checklist.pdf)

Agitation and pain scales

At times, it is helpful to utilize assessments or rating tools that assist clients and staff in identifying and rating an individual's level of agitation, aggression, or pain; the following are examples of assessment tools used for these purposes:

- Cohen Mansfield Agitation Inventory, Brief Agitation Rating Scale

- Richmond Agitation–Sedation Scale

- Berg Pain Scale

- Borg Numerical Pain Scale

All behavior has meaning. The information obtained from an assessment of cognition, agitation, and pain can be used in conjunction with information related to sensory processing to help create an SMP that targets the client's needs. According to the Agitation Decision Framework (Bidwell 2009), when people with dementia experience agitation, the assessment of potential triggers related to the physical environment or interactions with staff, other clients, or visitors is warranted. Once a potential trigger is isolated it can be addressed using direct interventions or environmental modifications, or by educating others in how to manage or avoid it. This process takes place in combination with the identification of both patterns of sensory processing that may also contribute to the client's agitation or pain and sensory-based supports.

After a short period of time spent implementing the interventions, re-assessment is used to determine their success in terms of helping to address the client's agitation, pain, and sensory-processing challenges. If problems in any of these areas continue, further assessment is necessary and the intervention planning and implementation process is repeated. The following recommendations have also been made for working with people with dementia, specifically when struggling with agitation, paranoia, or fearfulness (Doody *et al.* 2001):

- Spending time with the individual, providing reassurance and support

- Walking or other forms of light exercise (with supports as needed)

- Playing music (especially during meal times)

- Providing pet therapy

- Offering hand-holding or massage

- Adjusting the lighting

- Distracting the client

- Playing white noise or a sound machine at low volumes

- Organizing visits by family members during harder times of day to help ease transitions

- Providing simulated presence therapy (video- or audiotape recordings of a family member)

These recommendations are also sensory-based and incorporated into an individual's SMP. The SMP must be practical and readily available to everyone working with the individual.

To review, assessment is a necessary component of the SMP in order to provide the information necessary to decipher individualized needs, safety considerations, and goals, in order to create an individualized therapeutic plan. Multi-disciplinary professionals engage clients and caregivers in the evaluation and care planning process. Therefore, it is advantageous to use a team approach to gather the information needed to complete the assessment and screening processes. However, it must be within the professionals' scope of practice to assess each of the areas needed (safety and trauma considerations, agitation, pain, fall risk, balance, cognition, stage of dementia, sensory processing, medical, and other areas). Accordingly, the assessment process provides the evaluative information required to create each individual's SMP, and to provide the best possible care delivery both individually and programmatically for all clients.

Chapter 5

Sensorimotor Activities and Sensory-based Modalities

Everything we do and experience across the lifespan is sensory-based. Consider the sensory systems involved when looking at a book, listening to music, going through the movements necessary to get dressed, communicating with a loved one, and eating breakfast. Everyday activities require the experiencing and processing of sensory-based information from within the body and from the physical environment. The Sensory Modulation Program (SMP) aims to help people better understand each client's unique sensory integration and processing patterns, needs, and overarching goals so that they can use this information to strategically identify and tailor sensory-based supports as part of a comprehensive, individualized, intervention plan.

Each person has their own values, beliefs, strengths, and needs. Prior to offering sensory strategies it is important to identify the client's sensory integration and processing patterns, as well as their likes and dislikes, and the things they find comforting, interesting, and fun—or bothersome.

Whenever possible, observations of the person engaging with others, during various types of activity, in different environments (in addition to the use of more formal assessment tools), and at various times of day provides a wealth of information about what the person seeks, enjoys, dislikes, and avoids. While using a sensory lens, this information provides clues regarding potential types of sensory-based activity and modality the person may benefit from versus those that may be bothersome. How an individual responds to different situations, transitions, activities of daily living, and physical environments provides a rich representation of their sensory preferences and patterns. A more formal assessment process also contributes to determining the person's sensory preferences. Knowledge of the person's sensory preferences supports the ability to identify those sensory strategies that will be most effective. For more information on assessment, refer to Chapter 4.

The use of sensory strategies also requires the ability of the caregiver to recognize the signs of sensory overload, which is particularly important when working with vulnerable populations such as people with dementia. It is necessary to continuously assess for sensory overload in addition to what appears to be the "just right" amounts and types of sensory stimulation. The following are examples of signs to watch for that may indicate sensory overload. These include, but are not limited to, increases in or sudden onset of:

Neurophysiological changes:

- Sweating
- Dizziness
- Changes in balance
- Pallor
- Pupil dilation
- Yawning

Emotional and behavioral changes:

- Fearful responses
- Avoidance
- Irritability
- Anxiety
- Angry outbursts
- Aggression
- Agitation

Cognitive changes:

- Increased confusion

- Decreased orientation (time, place, self, etc.)

- Decreased attention span (more than typical)

Note: when any of these signs or symptoms appear it is important to stop using the particular sensory strategy until it is clear whether or not it is a contributor to the problem or if something else may be a factor. It is recommended that medical attention and guidance be sought in such a situation. This safety information must be kept in mind when introducing or using any of the sensory strategies explored in this book; medical and rehabilitation professionals involved in the care of the client should be informed of any additional safety considerations; and safety concerns should be noted in the client's medical record.

Calming and alerting strategies

Many people begin to expand their repertoire of sensory-based strategies by identifying the existing strategies they use to foster calming or alerting states and a combination of the two. Calming strategies are those that are soothing and induce a sense of safety, comfort, and relaxation, whereas alerting interventions exist on a continuum of being pleasant and uplifting to noxious (extremely bothersome). Most people intuitively understand why calming, sensory-based strategies would be desirable when working with people with dementia, but the rationale for the use of alerting strategies is less obvious. Alerting strategies are those that may be considered to be uplifting (cool drink, peppermint scent), a bit more intense (sour- or bitter-tasting foods, cool cloth to the face), or noxious (strong dislikes, different types of alarm to alert to a safety concern).

After taking an initial inventory of sensory-based strategies in the home or workplace, increasing the options available for both calming and alerting purposes is frequently the next step. While people have different perceptions of sensory input, and of what they find to be calming or alerting (or a combination thereof), Table 5.1 provides examples of common qualities of sensory input that tend to make the stimuli seem more calming or alerting.

Although people demonstrate unique preferences for and responses to sensory input, Table 5.2 provides examples of sensory-based strategies that are commonly considered to be further on either the calming or alerting ends of the continuum.

Table 5.1 Common qualities of calming and alerting stimulation

Calming	Alerting
• Familiarity	• Unfamiliarity or novelty
• Consistency	• Inconsistency
• Slow pace	• Fast pace
• Even, rhythmic beat	• Uneven beat
• Simplicity	• Complexity
• Low stimulus intensity	• High stimulus intensity

Table 5.2 Calming and alerting strategies

Calming	Alerting
• Hot shower/bath	• Cold or cool shower/bath
• Holding/stroking a pet	• Holding ice in hand or to face
• Warmth of a fireplace	• Being in a cool room
• Wrapping in a heavy blanket	• Wrapping in cool bed sheets
• Massage/deep pressure touch	• Fast-paced, upbeat music
• Isometric exercises/yoga	• Alerting sounds of nature (birds chirping)
• Leisurely walks	• Strong scents
• Slow/rhythmic music	• Light touch
• Calming sounds of nature (ocean)	• Aerobic exercise
• Humming/singing quietly	• Power walks
• Soothing scents (oils/lotions/candles)	• Rough or prickly materials/textures
• Soft materials/textures	• Fast or bumpy car ride
• Rocking in a rocking chair	• Spinning on a swing
• Swinging on a swing	• Fast and/or jerky movements
• Slow rhythmic motions (swaying to slow music)	• Bright or flashing lights
• Soft/low lighting	• Drinking tea or coffee
• Decaffeinated and herbal teas	• Biting into a popsicle
• Chewing gum, chewy or crunchy foods/candy	• Sour or hot foods/candy

Source: Adapted from Champagne (2011).

In addition to the use of strategies for calming or alerting purposes, it is also possible to use interventions to support a mixed response, such as having a calm body and an alert and focused mind.

When considering the use of sensory-based activities and modalities, in conjunction with any safety-related variables, the person's medical history, sensory tendencies, preferences, needs, and goals must be considered. For example, is the person sensitive to loud noises, sudden movements, changes in temperature, or certain types of tactile sensation? Does the person avoid specific kinds of stimulation and, if so, what kinds? Does the individual tend to seek out things to touch, hold, and interact with (the opposite of sensory sensitivity and avoiding)? What other kinds of stimulation does the person tend to seek out? When these questions can be answered, a list of strategies sorted by sensory systems will serve as a helpful resource to decipher other sensory-based strategies that can be used to increase or decrease different types of sensory input.

In addition to the *type* of stimulation an activity or modality affords, the intensity of the stimulation also plays a part in the perception of efficacy (Champagne 2011). Likewise, the time of day, how often, and how long it is used also play a role in the perceived degree of intensity experienced. The way in which sensory strategies are introduced and used also influences their efficacy. Furthermore, at different stages of dementia, a person's needs and preferences may change. For all of these reasons, it is important to remain attentive and continue to track how the person responds to the use of various interventions offered as part of the SMP.

Communication

In the earlier stages of dementia, an individual typically plays a highly active part in communicating their preferences for sensory-based and other therapeutic approaches. However, when the disease progresses and communication skills become increasingly more impaired, caregivers must play a greater role in understanding and communicating the person's preferences and needs. Remaining highly attentive to the more subtle signs of body language and other nonverbal signs of communication is necessary as the person's communication capacities change over time.

(Note: it is important to have [at least] a basic understanding of each of the sensory systems prior to use of sensory-based strategies and the SMP. Refer to Chapter 2 and the Resource section for more information and a review of the sensory systems and sensory integration and processing.)

Sensory strategies organized by sensory system

Once there is a general understanding of sensory integration and processing, and what tends to make things more calming, alerting, or some combination of both, many seek to develop a better understanding of the various sensory systems and how to use this knowledge more strategically. Initially, people (staff or caregivers) may want a list of the different kinds of sensory strategy (sensorimotor activities and modalities) sorted by sensory system to help increase their ability to recognize various strategies related to each sensory system. This desire tends to emerge in conjunction with the realization that a certain type of sensory input is preferred, sought out, or needed for any of a number of therapeutic reasons. The following list provides examples of common sensory strategies organized by sensory system. However, care must be taken when using this information. This list is provided to serve only as a guide and not as a protocol. Individualizing all sensory strategies based on the person's specific safety, sensory, medical, and therapeutic needs and goals is critical. Moreover, the overall experience of sensation is typically multi-modal.

While most people are aware of the five basic senses, there are actually eight:

- Tactile

- Proprioception

- Vestibular

- Visual

- Auditory

- Olfactory

- Gustatory

- Interoception

The tactile, proprioceptive, and vestibular systems are commonly referred to as the "powerhouses" because the "just right" amounts and types of input to these particular sensory systems (that is, perceived by the individual as desirable and safe) tend to decrease feelings of anxiety and agitation, and increase the ability to feel more organized, self-aware, and physically present. Although we will discuss the sensory systems individually, these three sensory systems are interconnected in several ways, and therefore also greatly influence each other.

Tactile system: touch

Tactile stimulation provides information about touch, pressure, pain, temperature, and vibration. The following list provides examples of objects, activities, and modalities that provide different types of tactile input:

- Art/craft supplies and activities

- Various types of yarns and fabrics

- Exploring different types of seeds and nature items

- Gardening activities

- Fidget items and stuffed animals (Figure 5.1)

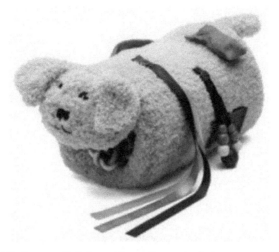

Figure 5.1 Twiddle Pup: stuffed dog with tactile manipulatives

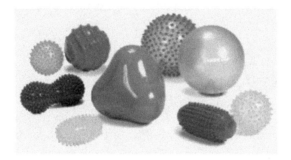

Figure 5.2 Assorted tactile fidget and stress balls

- Use of clay, play dough, different types of putty
- Kinetic or beach sand
- Cooking/baking supplies and activities
- Assorted types and textures of stress balls or fidgets (Figure 5.2)
- Soft blankets
- Soft and seamless clothing/socks
- Seating cushions
- Manicures/pedicures

- Hand-holding
- Use of lotions/powders
- Hand massage/body massage
- Hair brushing or body brushes
- Pillows
- Memory foam mattress pads
- Petting a cat or dog
- Puzzles
- Beanbags made with different types of bean and fabric
- Sorting and folding activities
- Fabric swatches on a large key ring (with assorted fabric types and textures)
- Lap quilts with many different tactile options to explore (Figure 5.3)
- Rolling yarn
- Items offering vibration (pillow, massager)
- Breeze from a fan, open window, or the wind outside
- Soft crocheted afghan, soft flannel, or cotton blanket
- Wall décor of different textiles woven into the theme of the art work (tiles, craft materials, fabrics)
- Guessing games: reach into a bag without looking and guess the different:
    - Nature items (pine cone, coconut, acorn)
    - Tactile qualities and shapes of items (e.g., soft/rough, round/triangular)
    - Types of fabric (cotton, flannel, denim, wool)
    - Types of coin
    - Types of hardware item and tool (screws, bolts, wrench, sandpaper)
- Pillows, lap pads, aprons, or bean bags with different objects to feel and identify

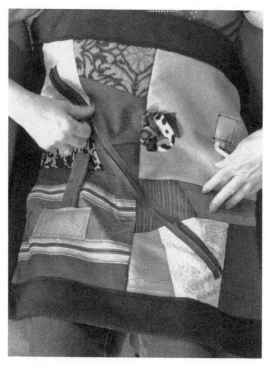

Figure 5.3 Lap quilt with tactile manipulatives

Generally, although people may have different responses, light pressure touch tends to produce more of an alerting response, whereas deep pressure touch tends to be more calming. Light pressure touch stimulation is produced when the tactile receptors that detect light touch pressure are activated. Some of the following activities and types of stimulation are examples of those that may trigger the light touch pressure receptors of the skin and corresponding responses:

- Being touched lightly
- Feeling light rain drops on the skin
- Being brushed up against lightly
- Stroking a pet lightly or stroking the skin lightly with fingers or a feather

Deep pressure touch stimulation occurs when the type of tactile stimulation experienced activates the deep touch pressure receptors. Some of the following activities and types of stimulation are examples of those that may trigger the deep touch pressure receptors of the skin and corresponding responses:

- Getting a massage (hand, neck, or body massage)

- Receiving a hug

- Using skin care supplies (creams, brushes, lotions)

- Feeling a weighted lap pad or shawl draped over the body

- Feeling of massage tools

Tactile hyper- and hypo-sensitivity

Hyper- and hypo-sensitivity patterns may be evident in any one or multiple sensory systems, including the tactile system. It is possible to experience tactile hyper-sensitivity (over-responsivity) and/or hypo-sensitivity (under-responsivity or difficulty in perceiving sensory stimulation) simultaneously because there are different types of tactile receptor. Tactile hyper-sensitivity is evident when a person experiences an adverse response to touch sensations that other people do not find bothersome or anxiety-producing. For people with hyper-sensitivity to tactile stimulation, being touched, sitting next to someone the client may come into physical contact with, the feeling of certain fabrics, having self-care activities performed, or even being hugged may be difficult to tolerate. When tactile hyper-sensitivities are evident, decreased tactile input and/or strategies to cope with touch sensations (e.g., during self-care tasks) can be helpful.

Tactile hypo-sensitivity is evident when it takes a lot more stimulation to notice or perceive tactile input than it would for most people. A lack of or a decrease in the awareness of touch, vibration, pressure, temperature changes, and/or pain can have a significant impact on safety, functional performance, and the ability to feel comforted. When tactile hypo-sensitivity is evident, increased tactile stimulation may support the capacity to register and notice tactile input that is comforting and organizing. Tactile input that may be useful to those with tactile hypo-sensitivity includes activities with more intensity or gradations of tactile stimulation (e.g., use of a recliner with vibration/massage options, sorting fabrics of varying textures, wrapping in a warm blanket). Additionally, tactile hyper- and/or hypo-sensitivities may emerge or be compounded by the progression of dementia. Thus, it is common to see tactile preferences change with the progression of dementia.

When implementing the SMP, the identification of the client's tactile preferences informs the ability to select and integrate the most supportive types of tactile-based intervention as part of the client's sensory diet. Ongoing observation and re-assessment of the sensory-based strategies being used will help to track whether the sensory diet interventions continue to be effective and when changes or discontinuation are warranted.

Proprioceptive system: body awareness, postural awareness, and movement

Proprioception is used in a therapeutic way by pinpointing activities and movements that can help a person feel more calm, oriented, coherent, bodily grounded, and self-aware, and support the ability to move the body. Activities that trigger the proprioceptive receptors include:

- Pushing/pulling activities
- Lifting and passing items
- Walking
- Isometric exercises
- Dancing
- Squeezing a stress ball
- Kneading dough or clay
- Stretching activities (such as tai chi, yoga, pilates) or exercises
- Playing active games (bowling, balloon volleyball), athletic activities (catch)
- Passing a weighted ball or other weighted item and trying to guess the weight
- Gardening activities (digging, planting)

Proprioception: hyper- and hypo-sensitivity
Hyper- and hypo-sensitivity to proprioceptive stimulation may exist for some individuals. Hyper-sensitivity to proprioceptive stimulation might be evident when a person demonstrates fearful or reflexive responses

to activities or input that trigger the proprioceptive receptors (muscles, joints, ligaments, tendons) during body-based movements, activities that require stretching or reaching, or pushing or pulling actions. Hyper-sensitivity to proprioceptive input may be evidenced when increased anxiety, avoidance behaviors, or stiffening of muscles occur during activities activating the proprioceptors.

Hypo-sensitivity to proprioceptive stimulation is evident when it takes a lot more stimulation to notice or perceive proprioceptive stimulation than it would for most people in the same age range. A lack of or a decrease in the awareness of proprioceptive stimulation can impact safety, movement, body and self-awareness, and functional performance. When hypo-sensitivity is evident, increased proprioceptive stimulation helps the individual to register and notice proprioceptive stimulation that is calming and organizing, and helps support movement. Hypo-sensitivity to proprioception may be evident when individuals demonstrate clumsiness or poor body awareness, or have trouble maintaining upright body positioning or difficulty sequencing their bodies through movement-based actions or activities.

Weighted modalities

One type of sensory-based modality that provides tactile and proprioceptive input, to varying degrees depending on how it is used, is a weighted modality. Weighted modalities are wearable items (vests, lap pads, blankets) or objects (dolls, stuffed animals) that have materials added to make them heavier. The heaviness of the item increases the amount of deep pressure touch and proprioceptive input for specific therapeutic reasons. Some of the benefits accruing from the use of weighted modalities with different populations include increased attention span, feelings of calmness and safety, greater body awareness, and improved rest and sleep (Champagne et al. 2015; Chen et al. 2013; Mullen et al. 2008). Figure 5.4 demonstrates a woman enjoying the use of a weighted quilt.

Which type of input is most activated when using different weighted modalities, deep touch pressure versus proprioceptive input, remains a subject for debate among professionals. When weighted modalities are used while standing or ambulating, both the deep touch pressure and proprioceptive receptors are recruited. The weight increases resistance to movement (proprioception) and also increases the deep pressure afforded to the skin (tactile) in the areas where the weight/deep touch pressure is applied. Depending on the intensity of the type(s) of movement the person engages in when using a weighted modality, there may be more or less proprioceptive and tactile input

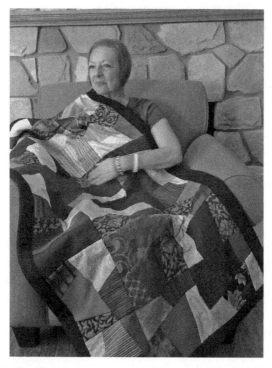

Figure 5.4 Weighted quilt

to the body (standing, walking, jumping, exercising). While sitting or lying down and using a weighted modality in a more passive manner, deep touch pressure receptors receive the bulk of the input, even though the proprioceptors are recruited to help the person change or maintain body position, or to shift or remove the weighted item (e.g., weighted blanket). Weighted modalities include:

- Dolls
- Stuffed animals
- Lap pads (weighted, gel; see Figure 5.5)
- Blankets
- Wraps/shawls
- Vests
- Belts

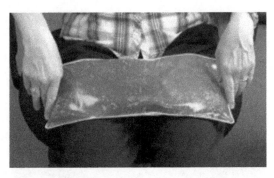

Figure 5.5 Weighted, gel-filled lap pad

When used with people with dementia, weighted modalities must be modified to accommodate for any and all precautions or safety concerns—or not used at all. Additionally, weighted modalities must never be used as a physical restraint. A physical restraint is something that cannot be easily removed at will, therefore the person must be able to easily remove and terminate use independently.

An assessment by a rehabilitation professional skilled in sensory integration and processing will help to identify the following: type(s) of weighted modalities to consider, amount of weight to use, amount of supervision required during use, any necessary vital signs or other types of monitoring, and a wearing schedule to ensure safe and effective use. Also, the type of weighting material used must be well contained, not easily removed or ingested, and washable, to minimize safety risks. Whenever there are safety concerns related to the use of a weighted modality, it is important to consult a medical or rehabilitation professional or obtain a physician's medical order and recommendations. While the use of weighted modalities is extremely helpful, their improper, unskilled, and unsupervised use has led to fatalities in vulnerable populations. Therefore, it is necessary to follow the safety recommendations reviewed.

Another way to obtain deep touch pressure input without the use of weight is through pressure-affording items or specialized garments such as compression socks, shirts/shorts, tank tops, lycra wraps, and/or blanket wraps. Like the recommendations outlined for weighted modalities, safety precautions must be taken to ensure the safe use and comfort of compression-affording items.

Vestibular system: balance, movement, and muscle tone

The vestibular system contributes to our sense of balance, body position, directionality, feelings of stability, bodily coordination, and muscle tone. The vestibular system informs us whether we are moving, if any of the things in our environment are moving, and about the direction and speed of these movements. A few examples of movement-related activities that provide vestibular input are:

- Walking

- Rocking or gliding in a rocker, recliner

- Stretching

- Making rhythmic movements or swaying

- Going up or down stairs

- Using the Wii

- Carrying out movement exercises from any position

- Dancing

- Playing balloon volleyball

- Bowling

- Playing target games (Figures 5.6 and 5.7)

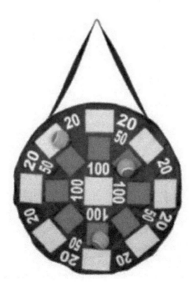

Figure 5.6 Dart ball game

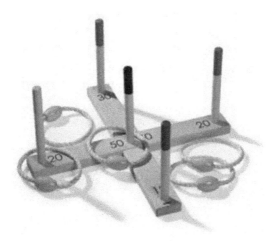

Figure 5.7 Ring toss target game

- Swinging

- Using therapy balls

- Changing positions or being transferred

- Riding in the car

- Doing tai chi/yoga

When providing interventions that increase vestibular input, care must be taken to avoid over-stimulating the individual, which may result in negative responses such as dizziness, headache, pallor, vomiting, and motion sickness. If someone is hyper-sensitive to vestibular stimulation it is particularly important to use vestibular input very cautiously. Vestibular hyper-sensitivity refers to difficulty tolerating movements that involve:

- Changes in speed (e.g., faster pace)

- Changes in direction

- Changes in body position (e.g., upside down versus right-side up)

- Lifting the feet from the floor during some activities (or positions)

- Uneven or unsteady surfaces

- A sense of disorientation after certain movements or changing body position

The severity of the hyper-sensitivity pattern also impacts the degree of movement a person will be able to tolerate. The more severe the hyper-sensitivity to vestibular input, the more over-stimulating and intolerable will engaging in different movements be, such as transfers, walking, or even rocking in a glider. When working with people with vestibular or movement hyper-sensitivities, encourage them to keep both feet on the floor (even when seated) and their eyes open; use activities that offer deep touch and proprioceptive input to help them feel more secure and bodily aware.

People with vestibular hypo-sensitivity need (and may even crave) more vestibular stimulation than other people in their age range in order to register and perceive vestibular information. Therefore, vestibular hypo-sensitivity frequently causes people to feel a strong desire for increased vestibular input, as seen in those who tend to pace, rock, swing, or seek out other types of movement. Providing multiple opportunities for safe movement throughout the day is important for people with vestibular hypo-sensitivity. Offering different types of seating option that do not pose a fall risk may also help, such as a BRODA glider rocker that automatically locks when a person stands to reduce their risk of falling.

Additionally, it is also possible for people to demonstrate different responses to various types of vestibular input, such as hyper-sensitivities to certain movements (tilting the head back to wash one's hair, bending over to put on a shoe) but also seeking out other types of movement. This combination of vestibular processing patterns is conceivable because of the functions of the different receptors of the vestibular system, the semicircular canals and otoliths. For more information on the vestibular system, refer to Chapter 2.

Caution: use additional caution with movement activities when people have problems with vision and/or balance and also during times of medication change.

Visual system: sense of sight

The visual system is the most complex of all the sensory systems, and it contributes to the ability to see and supports the visual, spatial, and perceptual ability to navigate in the world. The eyes are used to detect and transmit visual information about the world around us to the brain. The color, shape, size, contrast, depth, and placement of various objects, people, and other things in the environment are detected by the receptors of the visual system, and transmitted to the brain to integrate, process, and interpret. As people age, it becomes more difficult to see various contrasts, correctly perceive depth, and clearly discern certain colors (e.g., blue shades may look like green shades). Dark colors or patterns on the floor may be perceived as a barrier, and therefore the person may be fearful of crossing over or approaching it.

Visual stimulation is used for a variety of purposes, such as influencing a more calm or alert state. Although what is calming (or alerting) to one person may differ for another, the following list provides examples of visual strategies that may be used for either calming or alerting purposes:

Calming:

- Reducing lighting using a dimmer switch

- Providing soft, ambient, or colored lighting options

- Looking through books, magazines, or newspapers of interest

- Looking at pictures of nature scenes or animals

- Looking at pictures of activities or things the person previously enjoyed or currently enjoys doing (e.g., leisure, work, or family-based activities)

- Looking at pictures of places the person enjoyed being in or going to (e.g., home, vacation locations)

- Looking at a wind chime

- Looking at a mobile

- Looking at fish in a tank

- Looking at a waterfall

- Looking at a fire burning in a fire place

- Looking at projected images or scenes

- Seeing simple wall art

Alerting:

- Using bright colors (paint, lighting, décor)

- Using natural or bright lights (being cautious for glare/hyper-sensitivity to light)

- Displaying brightly colored, complex, or textured art work/posters

- Watching Hollywood classic movies

- Watching sports

- Playing balloon volleyball or target games (visual tracking is required)

- Watching a fast-paced dance performance

- Watching or interacting with a bubble lamp (with interactive switches)

- Using equipment with fiber optics, under supervision

- Using visual strategies with a variety of therapeutic aids, such as:

  - Matching games
  - Orientation boards (date, month, season, daily routine)
  - Wall murals or posters (environmental enrichment)
  - Map posters or large books of maps
  - Dark or colored sunglasses (to reduce glare or brightness in the environment)
  - Mirror (orient to self, use during self-care activities)
  - Family photographs (reminiscing)
  - Light therapy (e.g., overhead light adaptations, lamp, or light box), to support circadian rhythms, which are rhythmic biological cycles (e.g., sleep cycle)

Vision: hyper- and hypo-sensitivity

As with all of the other sensory systems, hyper- and hypo-sensitivity to visual stimulation may be evident, and to varying degrees, in people with dementia. Visual stimulation is a major part of the environmental stimuli that can impact how people feel and their behaviors over time. Identifying the types of visual stimulation that are most effective for different individuals throughout the course of the day is an important part of the SMP. Many people consider lighting and other elements of décor when determining the amounts and types of visual stimulation a person may experience, but few consider the amount of visual chaos and amount and intensity of visual stimulation experienced over the course of each day. At the same time, some environments do not offer enough stimulation, including visual stimulation. Finding the right balance for each individual, while taking into consideration unique sensory processing patterns, is key.

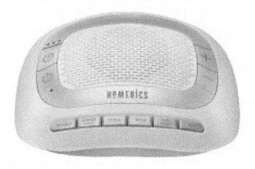

Figure 5.8 Sound machine

Auditory system: sense of sound

The auditory system supports the ability to hear all of the different types of noise and sound in the environment. The outer ear and the different receptors of the auditory system detect sounds and send auditory stimulation to the brain for further processing and interpretation. The following are general examples of strategies related to the sense of hearing that may be used as part of the SMP:

- Listening to music
- Using a sound machine (Figure 5.8)
- Listening to elements of nature (waves breaking on the shore, cat purring, birds chirping), talking books, videos/movies, singing
- Participating in sing-a-longs
- Being read to (newspapers, magazines, books, poetry, spiritual passages, etc.)
- Using a meditation bowl
- Whistling
- Playing an instrument (triangle, tambourine, piano, cowbell; see Figure 5.9)
- Following patterns or rhythms with the hands or hand-held instruments
- Playing listening games such as "name that tune"

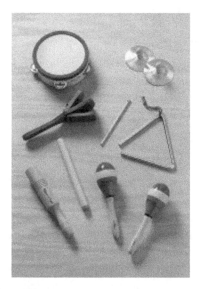

Figure 5.9 Musical instruments

- Engaging in a conversation

- Listening to music from specific eras, such as big bands, Frank Sinatra, Judy Garland, Elvis, Johnny Cash, Glen Miller, the Tommy Dorsey Orchestra, the Andrews Sisters, 1950s tunes

- Watching or listening to old comedy shows and films, such as those featuring Dean Martin and Jerry Lewis, Abbott and Costello, and Lucille Ball

- Using sound therapy equipment with a trained professional

Many people experience hearing loss when they age, while others may become more sensitive to auditory stimulation. Depending upon the person's auditory processing needs and preferences, it is important to modify the amount and intensity of auditory stimulation they experience, and to continuously monitor their response to auditory stimulation and also its cumulative effect. Interestingly, in a study by Locke and Mudford (2010), music was identified as a form of auditory input that decreased agitation and outbursts in people with dementia. A variety of research studies support the use of music with people with dementia (Blackburn & Bradshaw 2014; Cooke *et al.* 2010; Janata 2012; Lin *et al.* 2011; Vasionytė & Madison 2013). Further, a documentary called *Alive Inside* (details in the Resources section at the end of the book) provides case examples of how music is used to elicit a variety of positive effects in people with dementia.

Caution: too much noise, competing sounds, and loud or chaotic environments may have the effect of making a person with dementia feel disorganized, anxious, irritated, or agitated. Also, prolonged exposure to auditory stimulation may become overwhelming over time.

Olfactory system: sense of smell

The olfactory system detects chemicals, such as scents and smells, and has a direct connection to the limbic system (emotion center of the brain). Therefore, the sense of smell has a very direct and powerful influence on recalling memories and triggering emotions. Since the olfactory system has such a direct connection to emotions, it is necessary to be mindful of the different types of scent that are brought into the therapeutic environment. Aromas are commonly used therapeutically to achieve specific goals, such as triggering positive memories and emotions, fostering appetite, orienting to time/seasons/holidays, having a calming effect, and capturing attention.

Clinical aromatherapy involves using 100 percent essential oils for a specific therapeutic purpose. Recent research supports the skilled use of clinical aromatherapy with people with dementia (Press-Sandler *et al.* 2016). Given the high chemical make-up of essential oils, it is necessary to gain permission prior to their use in a healthcare facility. Most facilities do not allow the use of 100 per cent essential oils except by healthcare professionals with additional training or certification. Whether or not essential oils are used, a wide variety of olfactory stimulation options is available when working with people with dementia; for example, scented candles and soaps, and naturally smelling foods, plants, potpourri, herbs, and flowers. (It may also be necessary to have unscented items to hand should less stimulation be required.)

Similar to the other sensory systems, some scents tend to have a calming effect and others an alerting effect. Scents that tend to be calming include:

- Those that are familiar and pleasant

- Lavender

- Rose water

- Herbal teas

- Potpourri

- Chocolate

- Flowers

- Baby oil and powders

- Lotions and soaps

- Sandalwood

Scents that are often alerting include:

- Coffee

- Eucalyptus

- Peppermint or other types of mint

- Orange

- Grapefruit

- Cinnamon

- Perfumes/colognes

- Rosemary

- Pine

- Basil

Jars, baggies, or bottles containing items with different scents, scented bubbles, diffusers, plants (flowers, herbs, etc.), arts and crafts materials, scented art supplies (scented pencils or markers), and cooking or baking activities are used to introduce scented options as part of the SMP. Games in which individuals try to guess scents being presented to them can be fun, too.

Some people may be bothered by scents while others may have difficulty detecting olfactory stimulation as they age. Identifying any allergies, and assessing the person's olfactory capacities and degree of sensitivity to olfactory stimulation, is extremely important prior to introducing scented activities or modalities.

Caution: some individuals may be allergic or sensitive to certain scents, smells, or chemicals. Use olfactory stimulation with caution or not at all in these situations. Additionally, some facilities may not allow the use of scents that are not of a natural origin.

Gustatory system: sense of taste and oral motor functioning

The taste receptors of the gustatory system are chemical receptors called taste buds. Within the mouth there are also tactile receptors that help detect the textures and shapes of objects, foods, and liquids. In addition, proprioceptive receptors are involved in oral motor movements when we suck, chew, blow, or swallow. Considering the many ways in which the mouth receives and detects sensory stimulation helps determine which types of gustatory strategy to use to increase or decrease the amount and type of stimulation experienced. Examples of sensory strategies that involve the gustatory system include:

- Tasting activities or guessing games: different types of teas, herbs, different flavors of jellybeans, fruits, and ice creams/sorbets, etc.

- Blowing activities: bubbles, lightweight feather, through a straw into a drink

- Sucking: on a popsicle or thick liquids through a straw, hard candies

- Crunch or chew: popcorn, granola bars, crackers

- Daily tea times where a variety of teas are available

Caution: precautions may apply to people who have difficulty swallowing, have specific dietary needs, or respond negatively to certain textures. The use of straws must be monitored to assure that the person does not choke.

Interoceptive system: awareness of internal states

The interoceptive system allows us to recognize if we are feeling well, unwell, tired, or hungry, if we need to use the bathroom, have a pain, or are coming down with a cold. As dementia progresses, it becomes increasingly arduous for the person to be aware of these bodily processes and to verbally articulate them. Particularly during moderate or late stages of dementia, the person may have emotional or behavioral outbursts that can be an indicator of something happening internally that they perhaps cannot make sense of or articulate. It is always important to keep this in mind when working with people with dementia.

Indicators related to internal states—such as sleep/wake cycles; ability to eat (how much, how often, regularly or irregularly); conditions that may be causing discomfort or pain; medication changes; bowel or bladder problems; nausea—can be observed and used to target interoception interventions. All of these are indicators that at various times of the day the individual may feel discomfort or experience difficulty with everyday functioning. One of the ways in which sensory strategies are used to support interoception is, first, by identifying if any of these issues are occurring; second, alerting relevant medical professionals to ensure medically-based supports are in place; and third, offering sensory supports that might help to ease the difficulties or discomfort involved.

Sleep/wake cycles and eating or feeding challenges may be supported by closely inspecting the person's sensory diet to determine what additional supports may be helpful. When illness, bowel/bladder problems, or pain are suspected, working with a medical professional is necessary. Sensory supports when people are feeling unwell may include environmental or other strategies that make the individual feel safe and comforted.

The stress response is an internal state of distress, which becomes increasingly difficult to self-monitor and verbalize as the symptoms of dementia advance. Fearful or avoidant states are common signals that the person's stress response has been activated. Using the SMP to help the person feel safe, comfortable, cared for, and reassured is paramount to decreasing stressful and fearful responses, and potentially aggressive outbursts.

Multimodal multisensory experiences

So far, we have reviewed a variety of distinct sensorimotor activities and modalities according to each sensory system, but typically our experiences are multisensory in nature. While we can focus our attention on one or multiple senses, and we can reduce or block out the sensation from one or more sensory systems (close our eyes, wear ear plugs), human beings are continuously taking in and processing information from all of the sensory systems simultaneously. The following are examples of multisensory sensorimotor activities and modalities:

- Participating in an arts and crafts group
- Drawing while conversing with someone
- Cooking or baking
- Participating in a sensorimotor or exercise group
- Sitting in a rocking chair while watching a movie
- Grooming a pet while conversing with someone
- Planting or exploring a garden
- Sitting in or exploring a sensory room or sensory-enriched space

Table 5.3 Calming and uplifting strategies: sensory diet options

Sensory systems	Calming	Uplifting/alerting
Tactile (touch)	Warm blanket or sheet	Cool compress
Olfaction (smell)	Lavender or rose	Peppermint or rosemary
Auditory (sound)	Listening to instrumental music	Listening to upbeat music
Vision (sight)	Looking at pictures of family	Watching people dance
Gustatory (taste)	Cup of tea	Sweet foods/desserts
Movement (proprioception and vestibular)	Rocking in a glider rocker	Playing balloon volleyball
Interoception	Bedtime routine activities that foster sleep: • Dim the lights one hour before bedtime • Offer "sleepy time" tea • Provide a warm blanket while they sit in a rocker in their room prior to transfer to bed	Encourage the use of sensory-based, mindfulness activities that help to increase body awareness • Focus on the smell of a flower • Focus on the feeling of a weighted lap pad • Focus on the fish in a fish tank

Source: Adapted from Champagne (2017).

Over time, as the strategies that support calming or uplifting responses (or a combination thereof) become more apparent, it is helpful to create a document that is used to communicate this information with the different people working with the person, in addition to or as part of their sensory diet. Table 5.3 provides an example of such a document.

Such a communication tool can help inform loved ones and staff across different shifts about the specific sensory strategies that are helpful. This tool can also serve as a way to gather more information, as loved ones and staff from different settings (community-based programs) or across different shifts are asked to add to it as they discover additional supportive sensory strategies over time.

Chapter 6

Sensory Diet

Nothing revives the past so completely as a smell that was once associated with it. ~ Vladimir Nabokov

"Sensory diet" is a term created by occupational therapist Patricia Wilbarger (1995). A sensory diet is an individualized, daily routine that is strategically created to support safety, sensory needs, health, participation, and quality of life. In order to help clients and caregivers create a sensory diet, it is essential to first determine and list as many specific details about the person's daily routine as possible, as it typically occurs each week. Much of the time, creating a sensory diet begins by examining one typical day, or time of day, that may be particularly difficult and then expanding the focus to other times of day, additional days, and eventually the weekly schedule. Depending on the person, sometimes this process is fairly simple to complete and at other times may take much longer. Creating a sensory diet does require developing a relationship with the person, exploring past and current strengths and preferences, current needs, and triggers. Exploring sensorimotor activities, modalities, and environmental, and participation-related supports can also take time. Therefore, it is common to start with a basic sensory diet and to add to it as time progresses and other strategies are identified.

When the client is able to participate in the process of creating a sensory diet it is critical that they are central to the entire process. During the early stages of dementia people are very capable of contributing to all parts of this process, and they may or may not want loved ones or caregivers to be involved. In the moderate to late stages of dementia, as the person becomes less able to actively participate and communicate in the therapeutic process, seeking out caregivers or staff that are the most knowledgeable about the person is increasingly necessary. Through the use of direct discussion, phone calls, questionnaires, or other methods that do not violate any privacy rules or obligations, gathering information about the person's preferences supports the ability to individualize the sensory diet. While the client and caregiver(s) are central to the process, having an objective point of view of their needs after you are able to observe aspects of the daily routine lends valuable insights as well.

Creating a sensory diet is an exceedingly individualized and comprehensive element of the Sensory Modulation Program (SMP). Creating a sensory diet also entails completing or obtaining sensory-based as well as other assessment data (medical, rehabilitation), and engaging in the active exploration of different sensory-based approaches that are believed to be potentially helpful. All of the components of the SMP must be explored when creating and adapting a sensory diet over time. Some questions to consider asking when creating or modifying a sensory diet include:

- What are the person's sensory tendencies and patterns?

- What are the person's general likes and dislikes?

- What are the details of the person's daily routine and related helpful strategies versus triggers?

- What strategies tend to be calming and uplifting, and when are these strategies most helpful?

- What is distinct about the person's preferred strategies?

- What strategies help the person feel safe?

- What roles are/have been most important to the person?

- What are the person's previous and current leisure and social preferences?

- What strategies support the person's participation?

- What cultural and spiritual issues need to be considered?

If you will not be directly involved in helping to carry out the sensory diet, it is even more important that you work with those who will be otherwise what you help to create may not be valued or viewed as practical enough to use. Involving all relevant parties, whenever possible, is critical to the usefulness and implementation of the sensory diet.

Oftentimes, sensory strategies are considered or requested when there are increasing concerns about a person's safety, decompensation, sensory hyper-sensitivities, or sensory deprivation. The following sections consider some of the important aspects of safety, participation, and quality of life to bear in mind when creating a sensory diet with a person with dementia and involved caregivers.

Supporting safety, comfort, and participation

The sensory diet should include strategies that foster safety, comfort, and participation. These factors are important when trying to reduce the negative impact of dementia over time and to maintain the person's dignity, health, fitness, relationships, comfort, and safety. Offering activities that are related to meaningful and purposeful life roles and routines can help the person remain active and engaged. As the disease progresses, the person may go from being able to be largely independent and generally functional to needing more and more support to engage in the same activities and routines. The sections that follow provide examples of ways in which to support safety and participation in meaningful life roles and activities as people enter the moderate and later stages of dementia.

Supporting safety and relaxation

Helping the person with dementia feel safe and relaxed is not always easy. As dementia progresses, difficulty with confusion, fear, paranoia, feelings of loss and sadness, and many other variables contribute to the activation of the stress response. Using individualized, sensory strategies to prevent the person experiencing the stress response as much as possible, and also to address it when it occurs, is an important part of caring for a person with dementia. The following are examples to consider when trying to help a person feel more calm, safe, and relaxed:

- Music or music shows (radio, television, live)

- Comforting forms of touch

- Scents that are calming and soothing

- Herbal teas and other warm or cool drinks
- Pictures of loved ones that are easy to see (enlarged, within visual field)
- Furnishings that are comfortable (glider rocker, memory foam pad on mattress)
- Clothing that is comfortable (temperature, fit, type of fabric)
- Physical environment that is not over- or under-stimulating
- Adherence to all safety recommendations made by medical and rehabilitation professionals
- Daily activities that are engaging and modified to support participation at each stage of dementia
- Techniques to ensure quality sleep
- Baby dolls or stuffed animals
- Comfortable room temperature
- Activities or modalities to distract the person from that which is bothersome
- Novel experiences that are not triggering
- Techniques to help the person not feel alone
- Techniques to decrease fears and offer reassurance
- Regular contact with loved ones and caregivers
- Use of a weighted blanket or quilt with tactile manipulatives (Figure 6.1)

Supporting participation in self-care

In the moderate phase of dementia items needed for self-care routines should be set up for the person in a manner that is within their visual field and in the order in which they should be used. The person should perform those elements of the activity of which they are independently capable and help should be provided as needed (e.g., cues for next step, physical assistance, reassurance). Identification of how to best ensure success, comfort, and safety when completing daily routines is essential to quality of life.

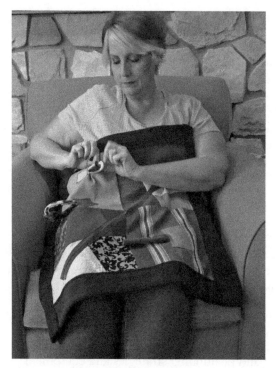

Figure 6.1 Weighted blanket with tactile manipulatives

Treating the person like the adult that they are while at the same time being compassionate, caring, and kind is very important.

As dementia progresses, eating and drinking independently becomes increasingly arduous. The creation of a dining environment that is pleasant, home like, and safe and supports a calm atmosphere is not always as easy as it sounds. Some of the things that can help to create such an atmosphere include:

- Seat people with hyper-sensitivities away from busy or more chaotic areas

- Leave plenty of room between people at each table; they should not be able to move into another person's space or touch their food

- Have loved ones or staff sit and eat with clients whenever possible

- Play soft, slow-paced, classical music, unless bothersome to some of the other people in the space

- Use chairs and seating supports that enable proper physical positioning

- Ensure that all items of food and drink are within the person's visual field and within reach so that they are not easily spilled

- Ensure anyone that needs toileting is not brought into the space until cleaned up so that odors related to hygiene needs are not present in the dining space (whenever possible)

- Set up the physical space so that it is pleasant, has home like décor, has noise reduction supports built in, and is functional for those using it

While people should remain as independent as possible, different strategies may become needed or useful over time. Working with a rehabilitation professional can help to identify feeding and adaptive equipment interventions that are safe and supportive, such as use of:

- Dycem mats to stop dishes and utensils from easily slipping when a person is trying to eat

- Seating and positioning strategies and equipment

- Different types of adapted utensils, cups, or dishware

- Strategies to support eating and drinking, or techniques for feeding people

- Problem-solving assistance when a person struggles with or is refusing to eat or drink

When the ability to swallow is impacted, it is necessary to obtain a referral for medical and rehabilitation services to assess and provide related services and recommendations.

Showering, bathing, taking care of one's hair, and other areas of hygiene are deeply personal and private, and impact self-identity and self-worth. At all times, respect for individuals' privacy needs and a comforting and caring approach to all aspects of care, especially personal self-care routines, are essential. At all ages, how we are treated is directly related to how we feel. Self-care is a significant part of everyone's daily routine and contributes to feeling like a meaningful, purposeful, and unique human being.

Having dementia does not have to be an experience that strips people of all dignity and self-respect. Self-care routines are one way in which to help the person demonstrate their own individual style (hairstyle, clothing) and feel refreshed, comfortable, and more alert each day. As dementia progresses, the amount and type of support needed to complete self-care routines increase. Being creative and compassionate helps the person to complete self-care routines in a way that is humane and holistic; for example:

- Use a pace that is supportive of the person's needs (moderate versus slow pace)

- Help them choose their clothing for the day or give them a choice of outfits to select from

- Never move or touch a person without greeting them (from the front, with eye contact, and in a caring manner) and talking to them about what you are going to be doing (taking them for toileting, bathing, dressing)

- Use a shower chair, hand-held shower, or whirlpool tub, if helpful

- Address trouble with balance or gravitational insecurity using some of the strategies identified as potentially helpful in Chapter 2

- Use a gentle touch when assisting with clothing changes

- Be attentive to and maintain privacy during all self-care routines

- Provide body and oral care options that are comfortable and preferred (favorite tastes, scents, and types [soaps, powders, lotions, oral care products])

- Ensure that undergarments, clothing, socks, and shoes are comfortable in fabric, type, and fit

- Offer manicures, pedicures, hairstyling options, as appropriate

Supporting rest and sleep

For most people the bedroom is a place of sanctuary, supporting rest, self-nurturance, peacefulness, and sleep. The quality of one's sleep is known to be critical to overall health and wellness. When people have dementia, and as the disease progresses, the ability to rest and sleep is frequently disrupted for a variety of reasons and increased support is needed to determine what strategies are most helpful. Sensory strategies can be used to support rest and sleep.

Considering that many older persons have various types of bodily aches and pains, strategies and supports that help manage pain and aid in rest and sleep should not be overlooked or minimized. While different seat cushions may be of concern to prevent bed sores and promote proper positioning, the type of mattress and mattress pad used sets the stage for the quality of a person's sleep and also for how the person's body will feel throughout the night and into the next day. Having a comfortable pillow and bed sheets is also key. Other sensory elements that influence the quality of sleep include:

- Room temperature

- Lighting that does not disrupt sleep

- Reduced noise in the bedroom and surrounding environment

- White noise, a sound machine, or a fan

- Access to sunlight during the day to help with regulating biorhythms

- Avoidance of technology use in the hours before bedtime

- Comfortable garments (e.g., fit, feeling of the fabric)

Sleep and wake cycles are important to pay attention to when trying to support quality sleep. To gently prompt waking up in the morning, alarm clocks that use a gradual increase in lighting or soft music can help make waking up in a routine way a more pleasant experience. Accessing natural light in the morning and witnessing the sun going down later in the day (bearing in mind visual sensitivities to light and glare) may help with the person's biorhythms. Light box therapy is another way to access light in the early morning to assist with biorhythms when natural light is not an option. Before using a light box, additional training and information is needed to fully understand what it entails and how to use it. If you are not a medical or rehabilitation professional, it is recommended that you seek guidance to ensure that light box therapy will actually be advantageous for the person you are working with.

Nutrition is another element that influences rest and sleep. Caffeine should be avoided for several hours prior to bedtime, which includes limiting access to coffee, tea, hot chocolate, and soda that contains caffeine.

Herbal tea or other drinks that are non-caffeinated can be used to help people relax before bedtime. In terms of food, the amino acid tryptophan is known for stimulating the neurochemical serotonin, and it is found in many foods (e.g., turkey, eggs, chicken, and nuts). Eating a dinner comprising foods containing this neurochemical has a calming effect, which can ease transition into the evening hours. Light snacks may be desired in the hours leading up to bedtime but avoiding foods that are spicy or high in fat content is recommended.

Supporting roles and social participation

Identifying the roles, vocations, and social activities that were meaningful to the person in the past and are relevant in the present provides a platform for brainstorming and deciphering activities, modalities, and environmental strategies that may be of interest. Consider the different sensory stimuli, activities, and meaning behind the various roles, work, and social activities the person enjoyed in the past and prefers in the present.

Below are examples of simple activities related to a person's previous vocation or hobbies that may be used with people with dementia (supervise the use of small or sharp objects and ensure all items are used safely).

Early or moderate dementia:

- Actively engage in leisure and work-related activities that continue to tap into work and leisure interests from the past: gardening, going to the movies, visiting friends and family, exercising, cooking and baking, building a birdhouse and feeding/watching the birds, going for walks, playing games (cards, bingo), etc.

- Actively engage in puzzles, crafts, guessing games, looking at magazines, watching movies or television shows, taking field trips to places that are related to prior vocations and hobbies

- Ask people questions about their past work and leisure interests or ask them to describe to others what they did for work or enjoyed in their free time (with or without the support of loved ones, as appropriate)

- Discuss trivia from the era related to past social norms, work, and leisure activities and discuss comparisons to present day norms

During moderate stages of dementia, sorting and other kinds of exploratory or repetitive activities may be of interest to the person if related to prior work or leisure interests. The following are examples that have sensory-related elements as well as meaning and purpose:

- Seamstress: sorting packets of sewing patterns, buttons, fabric types or shapes

- Carpenter: sorting different types of small, safe hand tools, sanding activities, looking at pictures related to carpentry

- Car mechanic: sorting car keys, bolts, washers, or screws, looking at pictures of different types of cars and parts of car engines

- Writer: providing a basket with pens, pencils, a notebook, and dictionary and suggesting some writing activities

- Homemaker: sorting socks, folding clothes, flipping through a cookbook, looking through a family photograph album

Supporting fitness and leisure participation

People with dementia should have access to safe and comfortable forms of movement to maintain fitness and prevent deconditioning (Chang *et al.* 2011; Lee *et al.* 2016; Rolland *et al.* 2007). For instance, a six-month walking program was found to support cognition and performance in activities of daily living in clients with Alzheimer's (Venturelli, Scarsini, & Schena 2011). Another study revealed that people with Alzheimer's engaging in a community-based exercise program demonstrated increased functional ability (Vreugdenhil *et al.* 2012).

While research supports the benefits accruing from movement and exercise for people with dementia, there are many safety variables to consider when working with this client group. Since people with dementia often have other medical conditions and requirements, consultation with medical and rehabilitation professionals to ascertain the safety precautions to follow when engaging people in movement-based activities and exercises is important. Organizing casual leisure activities that the client enjoys is one way in which to engage them in active movement, which is an essential part of a sensory diet (Fenech & Baker 2008). The following are common activities used to promote movement in people with dementia:

- Target games, such as balloon volleyball, ring toss, mini-golf, bowling

- Gardening activities

- Cleaning activities

- Exercise and stretching routines from a seated position

- Walks

- Modified yoga or tai chi

- Dancing

- Passing and guessing the weight of a weighted ball or stuffed animal

- Waving scarves, ribbons, pom poms, or streamers during movement

- Playing games, such as checkers, chess, cards, bingo

- Using the Wii

Following safety precautions, including providing the amount and type of support and supervision needed at all times, is required when engaging in movement-based activities or exercises to prevent falls and respond to other medical and safety concerns.

Individual and programmatic applications

Sensory diets can be created and used on both an individual and programmatic basis. They can be tailored to one individual's routine and sensory needs or designed to meet the needs of an entire group's SMP. Close observation of daily and weekly routines is necessary in order to create a sensory diet suited to the needs of the intended individual or group. Providing visual cues and reminders for the date, weather, daily schedule, and holidays all help people feel more oriented and able to anticipate the next activity or understand the expectations of the SMP. In order to prevent sensory deprivation, even those in the middle and late stages of dementia must have comfortable opportunities for engagement in programming. With an emphasis on sensory-based strategies and sensory diet, attention to sensory supports ensures that people at all stages of dementia have sensory-enriched, safe, and comfortable opportunities to participate in the daily routine to the best of their ability.

Sensory diet communication

The consistent implementation of a client's sensory diet is enabled through documentation and communication of the preferred sensory-based strategies that are integrated into the daily routine. There are many ways to inform others about a client's sensory diet, including:

- Document details in the client's medical records

- Create a checklist to be used by the client and staff on each shift

- Provide a visual schedule using pictures or words

- Input details on an Excel spreadsheet

- Create sensory diet guides based on cognitive ability level (Champagne 2011)

Another way in which to ensure that a sensory diet is consistently implemented is to ensure that items needed to apply the person's sensory-based strategies are organized and readily available. Using baskets, bins, and organizers helps keep items from being lost or disorganized.

In summary, the concept of the sensory diet has grown significantly since its inception. Like the SMP, a sensory diet is created and used on individual and programmatic scales. Being mindful and creative about the daily routine and the integration of sensory-based strategies that help people feel safe and able to participate is paramount when working with people with dementia. When using sensory diets in a skilled manner, the consistency and individualized interventions integrated into the daily routine ease transition times and foster quality of life.

Chapter 7

Environmental Modifications and Enhancements

The environment must be rich in motives which lend interest to activity and invite the [person] to conduct his own experiences. ~ Maria Montessori

People with dementia have sensory-based needs that differ from those of other populations. In order to adequately identify and implement supportive modifications and enhancements, people with dementia benefit from a sensory focused assessment of the physical environment in which they live. Many resources, such as home modifications and adaptive equipment, address the physical challenges and needs of people who have experienced a stroke or other types of traumatic injury or disease, or have dementia. While such modifications and equipment are important, less information has been published on the sensory-based, environmental needs of people with dementia. Thus, the purpose of this chapter is to explore sensory-based environmental modifications, enhancements, and equipment commonly used with people with dementia.

Enabling and empowering environments

Whenever possible, the environmental design of spaces for people with dementia must have a primary focus on empowerment, safety, functionality, and enablement of those who will use them. To meet this goal, it is important to take into account some of the following client and environmental considerations when designing such spaces:

- Safety needs

- Functionality

- Range of cognitive abilities of the users

- Range of sensory processing needs of the users

- Medical and physical issues

- Social participation challenges

- Cultural considerations

- Spiritual considerations

A variety of design qualities are promoted as important when designing spaces for people with dementia, and homelike décor is commonly cited. This involves safe furnishings, and pictures and other items that stimulate memories, increase curiosity, and draw attention to the environment.

Due to the inevitable decrease in cognitive ability and spatial orientation that occurs with dementia, the floor plan is a key element of environmental design (Marquardt 2011). Simple floor plans within main living spaces that are easily seen and navigated without the need for signage enable individuals to navigate space and find their way (*ibid.*).

Functionality within the space is critical, as is providing the equipment necessary to ease and comfort those engaging in activities of daily living, social and leisure activities, mobility, and movement opportunities (e.g., dining, bathing, dressing, ambulation). In order to design spaces that provide comforting experiences for people with dementia, who have a variety of sensory processing, physical, and cognitive needs, everything from lighting, adaptive equipment, furnishings, space configuration (floor plan, placement of furniture, and décor), use of color (color schemes should not be too bright or too light), sound dampening, and a variety of other homelike elements must be considered.

Homelike environments

A homelike environment is one that does not feel institutional but instead is cozy, and provides comforting and familiar stimuli (Victoria State Government 2017). A homelike environment in a hospital or other type of medical, skilled nursing, or mental health setting is typically created by:

- Ensuring a welcoming atmosphere
- Following an individualized approach
- Facilitating meaningful relationships (e.g., with family, friends, clergy)
- Using client first language
- Observing cultural, religious, and spiritual customs
- Encouraging active engagement in activities of daily living
- Designing a smaller scale living environment than is usual in clients' own homes (easier to manage and navigate)
- Providing home like furnishings in both indoor and outdoor spaces (e.g., kitchen, dining areas, bathrooms, gardens)
- Personalizing bedroom spaces
- Using warm colors
- Dampening sound with drapes, wall hangings, wall or ceiling panels
- Ensuring freedom of movement (continuous indoor and outdoor spaces)
- Promoting individual control and decision making, whenever possible
- Maintaining a flexible management and supervisory approach
- Using unobtrusive equipment and devices
- Offering a wide range of sensory-based activity and experiential opportunities
- Maintaining an organized environment (not chaotic or cluttered)

In addition to the recommendation of creating a homelike environment, other practical environmental adaptations and equipment recommendations are:

- Placing items within individuals' visual fields (e.g., food, activities, television)

- Providing furnishings that are comfortable and do not contribute to fall risk (glider rockers that lock in place when a person stands)

- Putting names and personal items on bedroom doors to support room recognition (e.g., picture of person and family)

- Using dining room tables that allow for wheelchair arms to fit underneath

- Offering different lighting options (lamps, dimmer switch, low tech illumination devices, natural or full spectrum lighting rather than florescent lighting)

- Providing clothing display hangers or hooks

- Providing adaptive equipment (e.g., weighted utensils, adapted cups/plates, walkers)

- Providing specialized bathroom equipment (e.g., raised toilet seat, tub bench, hand-held shower, grab bar, anti-slip mat or decals in shower/bathtub)

- Providing an adapted bathtub (built-in tub bench, multiple water jets, and a side entry doorway to prevent falls)

- Using heat lamps in bathing areas

- Using a blanket warmer

- Providing comfortable items necessary for postural support (e.g., seat cushions, chair pads)

- Providing bedding and mattresses that are sensitive to individual preferences

- Removing small items that may become choking or fall hazards

While people with dementia do demonstrate some common sensory-based patterns, nonetheless everyone is unique. For instance, most people do not enjoy glare from the sun shining in through bare windows (without curtains or blinds), but some people may want to be able to look out the window or go outside and experience natural light. Differences in sensory processing needs make it challenging to create or modify environments serving more than one person, yet attention must be paid to the balance between physical environments that are overstimulating and sensory depriving. Flexibility in the design of spaces and equipment available is essential in order to adapt the environment to support different needs. Several people talking, overcrowding in certain areas, alarms, loud singing, clapping, and higher television volumes are examples of sounds that may become overwhelming to some individuals. At the same time, some clients may be hearing impaired and need the volume to be set louder in to order hear. This is just one example of why it is essential to create and modify spaces that can be adjusted to the changing needs of the client population being served. Overstimulation and sensory deprivation both negatively impact cognitive ability, overall health, quality of life, and behavior of people with dementia.

Many organizations providing services to people with dementia work hard to make main living spaces homelike in décor and to also offer spaces dedicated to other activities (e.g., activity and movement groups, larger gatherings, arts and crafts, gardening). Adding sensory enhancements such as aquariums also helps to increase satisfaction for clients and staff alike (Edwards, Beck, & Lim 2014). In addition to homelike spaces, over the last 60 years "sensory rooms" have become increasingly popular for use with people with dementia in skilled nursing care facilities.

Sensory rooms

Sensory rooms are specifically designed to offer enhanced opportunities for safe, sensory-enriched experiences. Sensory room is a broad term encompassing a wide range of provision. Currently, sensory modulation rooms, sensory integration rooms, Snoezelen® or multisensory environments are the most commonly found types of sensory rooms discussed in the literature (Champagne 2011), and sometimes a combination of sensory room types is created and used. Until recently, multisensory environments (based on Snoezelen®) were the most common type of sensory room used with people with dementia in skilled nursing or other long-term care settings.

Multisensory environments

Multisensory environments (MSEs) are artificial environments specifically designed for and used with a wide variety of populations, including people with dementia. The initial MSEs were created in the 1970s in the Netherlands, at the De Hartenberg Centre, and were initially known as Snoezelen® rooms (Hulsegge & Verheul 1986). The term Snoezelen® evolved from the Dutch term "snufflin," which means to smell and doze (*ibid.*). The design of these spaces was significantly influenced by the disco era, and some of the technology that evolved during that time period is still used today. The word Snoezelen® was originally chosen because the initial

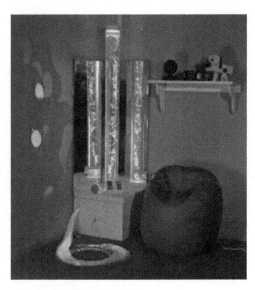

Figure 7.1 Multisensory environment equipment

goals of sensory rooms were to provide a safe, therapeutic environment offering specifically tailored and sensory-rich opportunities for people with severe and profound dementia and intellectual and developmental disabilities (*ibid.*). Various types of seating (large recliners, chairs, and different types of vibrating mat), light sources (projectors, different colored lighting), and interactive switches to operate items in the room are a few examples of the different kinds of equipment used in MSEs. People with more severe and profound diagnoses tend to have difficulty with cognition, sensory processing, self-regulation, and participation in everyday activities, and are apt to become easily overwhelmed by the intensity of stimulation provided by most natural environments. For these reasons, Snoezelen® was designed to provide the ability to easily control and vary the amount and type of stimulation offered by each piece of equipment, and to provide interactive options that meet the needs of each client (*ibid.*). Over the years, the term Snoezelen® was patented and, as a result, these spaces began to be referred to as multisensory environments (MSEs). Figure 7.1 shows types of equipment often used in MSEs.

When used in a traditional way, the general types of equipment contained within MSEs include:

- Bubble columns (with or without interactive switches, different color lighting options, plastic fish that float within the bubble lamp)

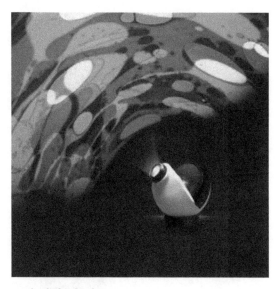

Figure 7.2 Projector for light displays

- Fiber optic equipment

- Different seating options (vibrating mats/chairs, large and supportive hammock-like chairs, bean bags, water beds/chairs)

- Stereo equipment

- Aromatherapy equipment

- Interactive switches contained within stuffed animals or control boards

- Projectors (projecting color swirls or images [stationary or rotational]; see Figure 7.2)

The equipment must be set up in a way that is safe and functional and affords a great deal of flexibility for offering and managing the amount and types of multisensory stimulation the space provides.

Increasing the amount of stimulation to help target a client's goals, needs, and preferences can be achieved in several ways: turning on more than one piece of equipment at a time, raising the volume, increasing the lighting, creating wall spaces with different manipulatives (Figure 7.3), and providing more opportunity for active participation.

To decrease the amount of stimulation, the converse is true: turn off some of the equipment, lower the lighting, reduce the volume, use one

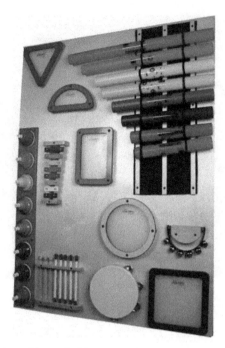

Figure 7.3 Wall hanging with musical instruments

piece of equipment at a time, take a slower paced approach, and make activities less challenging. The amount and type of stimulation provided are based on the sensory preferences and therapeutic goals of the individual, including the particular amount and types of stimulation they like. During the early years of Snoezelen®, its overarching goals were typically to offer the client:

- Choice of and control over environmental stimuli

- Environmental exploration and interaction

- Opportunities for relaxation

- Leisure and social participation

Over time, the use of MSEs has expanded and these goals continue to be valued but individualization is key! The MSEs are now also used with a wide variety of clientele with many distinct needs and goals. Some examples of various populations and settings that currently use MSEs are:

- Children with learning and developmental challenges in school settings

- Veterans living in long-term care hospitals

- People residing in short- and long-term mental healthcare facilities

- People with intellectual or developmental disabilities attending community-based day programs

- People of different ages and abilities living at home

- Older persons living in nursing care facilities (with and without dementia)

Many studies have investigated the efficacy of Snoezelen® and MSEs with people with dementia, as well as other populations. Recent studies on the use of MSEs with people with dementia reveal positive results (Baker *et al.* 2003, 2011; Bera 2008; Chung *et al.* 2002; Cox, Burns, & Savage 2004; Hope 1997; Hope & Waterman 1998; Maseda *et al.* 2014a, 2014b; Milev *et al.* 2008; Riley-Doucet 2009; Sánchez *et al.* 2013; van Weert *et al.* 2004), including:

- Physical outcomes: positive changes in balance, heart rate, and oxygen concentration

- Agitation: decreased agitation, restlessness, wandering, and aggressive behavior

- Mood-related outcomes: increased happiness, less boredom and negativity, decreased depression and stress

- Cognitive outcomes: improved cognition, active and alert behaviors

- Communication: increased response to speaking, talking in full-length sentences, increased ability to relate to others

- Participation: increased participation in activities of daily living, and greater interaction during activities

Figure 7.4 shows two women socializing in a multisensory environment.

Sensory integration rooms

In addition to multisensory environments, there are sensory integration rooms. A sensory integration room is a type of therapeutic space created and used in a manner that is specific to the Ayres Sensory Integration (ASI®) fidelity criteria, by rehabilitation professionals skilled in ASI®

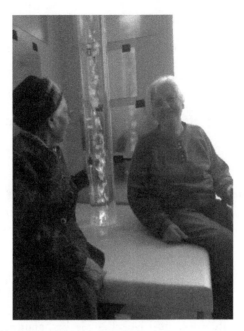

Figure 7.4 Socializing in a multisensory environment

(Parham *et al.* 2011). Sensory integration rooms contain mats and climbing, suspended, and other forms of equipment, used to foster active movement, self-awareness, and participation within the context of play, leisure, and social engagement (e.g., exercise balls, swings, climbing equipment, ball pit). The ASI® approach is used for very specific assessment and therapeutic purposes and is not to be used by caregivers or professionals for whom ASI® is not within their scope of practice. Generally, rehabilitation professionals (occupational therapists, physical therapists, speech and language pathologists) are the most common professionals providing ASI® as a therapeutic approach for people of all ages facing sensory integration challenges that make engaging in daily life roles, routines, and activities challenging.

Sensory modulation rooms

Sensory modulation rooms (SMRs) are created and used by a variety of interdisciplinary professionals, caregivers, and clients who have received training on the subjects of sensory modulation theory, supporting neuroscience, and techniques (Champagne 2011). Training is necessary to support the safe, skilled, and responsible use of sensory modulation-related approaches. Sensory modulation rooms are decorated according to a specific theme or can be home like in nature, with age-appropriate furnishings and therapeutic options that are used to help people meet their therapeutic goals. A SMR is frequently used to promote feelings of safety, comfort, self-regulation, engagement in coping, leisure, and social activities, and the use of therapeutic activities and equipment addressing different sensory processing-related needs and goals.

As explained in Chapter 2, sensory modulation is the regulatory component of sensory processing, thus SMR spaces are those that contain the décor, furnishings, and items that can be used for calming, alerting, comforting, and nurturing purposes. Since SMRs are created and used in a wide variety of settings, the design of each space must follow all regulations and safety considerations specific to each site. Safety considerations will differ depending on each organization. Therefore, it is important to work with the leadership of each organization when designing SMRs to ensure adherence to all organizational policies, procedures, and safety requirements.

When creating SMRs for adolescents, adults, or older adults, some of the common furnishings and equipment contained within the spaces are:

- Different types of seating (rocking chair [Figure 7.5], glider rocker, large bean bags, recliners, massage chairs, comfortable couches)

- A lockable cabinet or closet

- Projectors

- Fish tank, waterfall, or bubble lamp

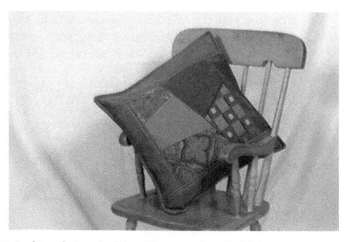

Figure 7.5 Rocking chair and pillow with assorted tactile fabric options

- Aquarium
- Stereo system
- Musical instruments
- Sound machine
- Wall art (pictures, tactile wall hangings, murals)
- Carpeting
- Window treatments
- Dimmer switch
- Mobile
- Art supplies
- Books, magazines, self-help books
- A book shelf to help keep things organized
- Weighted modalities (lap pad, dolls, stuffed animal)
- Gel-filled lap pads (with or without items inside; see Figure 7.6)
- Bins labeled by sensory system, containing corresponding items
- Bin labeled "used items" to put items in after use for cleaning

Unlike other types of sensory room, it is encouraged that each SMR is named according to its theme or goal(s) for use, such as the serenity room, zen room, chill ville, oasis space, comfort room, sensory exploration space, and so on (Champagne 2006, 2011). Sensory modulation rooms

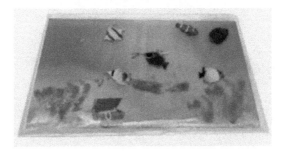

Figure 7.6 Gel-filled lap pad

were initially created to provide a sensory-enhanced sanctuary for people receiving mental health services, and are now being implemented across a variety of settings, including:

- Skilled nursing facilities
- Schools
- Acute inpatient psychiatric units
- Hospital emergency departments
- Long-term care settings
- Veterans' hospitals
- Partial hospital programs
- Community-based programs
- Forensic settings
- Home-based settings
- Outpatient settings
- Staff lounges

Some of the typical goals of SMR use are, among others, fostering feelings of safety, relaxation and comfort, self-soothing, distraction, self-regulation, leisure or social participation, sensory integration and processing skills, mindfulness practice, and various therapeutic approaches supporting the recovery process.

Sensory supportive enhancements for the *whole setting* are also important, and practically achieved by increasing safe, sensory-supportive options offered in each space as renovations are made over time, and also when planning different building projects. The ongoing effort to consider ways in which to implement sensory enhancements and modifications across each space within each setting is part of an international culture shift to provide more nurturing and healing environments of care (Champagne 2011).

Sensory carts

Sensory carts make SMR options mobile! Sensory carts provide the ability to keep sensory strategies organized and bring them to individuals' rooms, group sessions, day rooms, offices, sensory room spaces, and much more. Sensory carts may be organized in some of the following ways:

- Themed cart stocked with items that are related to a particular theme: sleep cart, self-care cart, gardening cart, sensory modulation cart, activities cart

- Multipurpose cart offering a variety of safe activity and commonly used items in order to make them more easily accessible

- Snoezelen®/MSE style cart offering a projector, fiber optic spray, bubble tube

- Stages of dementia cart, organized such that items appropriate for people at moderate stages of dementia are in one area and options more appropriate for people at later stages are contained in another

- Lockable cart for items that may have safety concerns or require close supervision in use

In most hospital, medical, forensic, and skilled nursing facilities, policies and procedures are developed for MSEs, sensory modulation rooms and spaces, and sensory carts to ensure their safe and skilled use and maintenance.

Sensory kits

When working with people with dementia, it can be helpful to have a sensory kit containing sensory-supportive items that are specific to the individual's sensory needs, likes, and therapeutic goals (Champagne 2011). In addition to sensory carts, a sensory kit provides an organized place in which to keep each client's preferred items more easily available to them anytime, anywhere! Many distinct types of container are used to make sensory kits, such as boxes, bins, large pocketbooks or beach bags, suitcases on wheels, or anything that is functional, and easy to clean and replace. A sensory kit makes it easier for staff and loved ones to have items that are helpful to the person on hand. Whenever possible, have the client and involved family members help create the sensory kit and identify items that may be preferred.

In addition to individualized sensory kits, sensory kits suitable for programmatic applications are also helpful and used for similar reasons (when running groups, during down time, when clients are in need of an activity or certain type of stimulation).

Like sensory carts, sensory kits can also be organized thematically, for example:

- Nature kit: pictures of nature scenes, containers with different items from nature (pine cone, rosemary sprig, shell, bird seed), nature or gardening magazines

- Holiday or seasonal kit: holiday or seasonal pictures or magazines, decorative items from the varied holidays or seasons, CDs with music related to the season, holiday recipes, related coloring books or simple crafts

- Memory box: personal items relevant to an individual's life (vocational, family, leisure, personal items that are not going to be problematic to lose)

- Sports basket: baseball or other sports cards, pictures of famous athletes, equipment related to different sports, sports videos or recordings, sports-related trivia books

- Reminiscence box: items, trivia books, pictures, or videos related to the era during which the persons in care were young

- Self-care box: items specific to the likes of the individual, such as roll-on scents, special brush, sachet with favorite dried herbs, preferred massager, favorite lotion, daily reflections book, CDs of favorite relaxation music

- Pet care box: pictures of pets, items used to groom a pet, magazines and videos of cats, dogs, birds, and so on

- Vocational box: safe tools, pictures, videos, books, magazines related to different vocations (carpenter, mechanic, nurse, homemaker)

- Spiritual kit: spiritual books, rosary beads, hymns, other items related to beliefs, spiritual recordings or videos

- Doll care kit: doll, doll clothes, furniture, receiving blanket, bottle, and other related items

- Tool kit: a variety of tools that are safe enough to have available to the persons exploring them

- Sorting kits: items that are safe in size and can be sorted, such as very large buttons, socks, different types or shapes of fabric, strips of yarn, baseball and playing cards, face cloths, large beads (items must not pose an ingestion risk for individuals who put things in their mouth [common in moderate to late stage dementia])

When creating sensory kits, being creative and providing items that can be used safely are paramount. For instance, if the person is not safe with small items (ingestion concerns) then larger items are necessary. It is also best to avoid using items that if lost would pose a significant problem for one reason or another (expensive or irreplaceable items, such as jewelry). Safe and supervised use is key to success, to ensure the person does not get hurt or overstimulated, or become bored when using the sensory kit and its contents. Determining and keeping the sensory kit in a specific location is necessary to ensure safe use and access when desired.

Sensory gardens

Sensory gardens are also sensory modulation-type spaces that capitalize on the use of the natural environment for therapeutic purposes. In addition to creating sensory gardens outdoors, it is also possible to bring elements of the natural environment indoors (indoor herb, vegetable, or flower gardens). Asking for and integrating the client's ideas and preferences as part of the sensory garden planning process is greatly encouraged. Additionally, be sure to avoid plants or items that may have an adverse effect on users, such as those causing an allergic reaction. Whenever appropriate, the client's safe and active involvement in all stages of sensory garden development is advantageous.

What makes a sensory garden different from a traditional garden? Sensory gardens are specifically created and used with the goal of enhancing the sensory-based options available to clients. During its creation and maintenance over time, there is also an intentional focus on including the items, elements, and furnishing that target the different senses. Some examples of different items and equipment that might be part of a sensory garden are provided below, categorized by sensory system:

- Sounds: plants that make a noise when wind passes through (bamboo, tall grasses), wind chimes, waterfalls, fountains, ponds, plants and garden items that attract wildlife safe for the client population (birds, butterflies, hummingbirds), outdoor instruments, music.

- Smells: aromatic plants and herbs (e.g., mint, rosemary, basil, sage, lavender, lilacs, geraniums, roses). Plants must be spaced so that scents are not overwhelming and to permit access that will help people more easily identify each scent. Plants that are poisonous to ingest must be placed well out of reach.

- Sights: plants that have different colors and textures (leaves, blooms, barks), and attract butterflies and hummingbirds are commonly enjoyed. Equipment targeting the sense of vision may include bird feeders, sculptures, fountains, or ponds. Provide shaded as well as sunny areas, and different seating options.

- Tastes: edible plants (fruits, herbs, mints, spices), water fountain.

- Touch: plants of different textures (lamb's ear, moss, cat tails, ferns). Garden options that promote interaction (instruments, safe plants and water options within reach), safe gardening tools, areas for interaction with soil/planting, and equipment making it possible for clients to assist in watering the plants.

- Movement: pathways that foster safe ambulation and wheelchair accessibility. Circular or figure of eight paths help decrease wandering to unsafe or distant locations. Interactive opportunities, such as labyrinth, outdoor instruments, different seating options, gliders or swings (if safe for the client group).

Caution: consider the safety needs of all those who will use the garden and be aware of allergies and any medical concerns. Avoid poisonous, spiny, and thorny plants and always provide supervision when using sensory gardens and the contents therein.

There are many research studies supporting the positive effects of indoor and outdoor gardening, and other outdoor activities, with people with dementia (Calkins, Szmerekovsky, & Biddle 2007; Connell, Sanford, & Lewis 2007; Detweiler & Warf 2005; Gigliotti & Jarrott 2005; Gonzalez & Kirkevold 2014; Grant & Wineman 2007; Hernandez 2007; Jarrott & Gigliotti 2010; Lee & Kim 2008; Murphy *et al.* 2010).

In summary, providing enhancements and modifications to physical environments is one of the major components of the SMP. The amount and type of stimulation a physical environment affords are strategically used to foster feelings of safety and the ability to function, and to maintain health and quality of life for as long as possible. There are several options for home use and for implementation across a variety of different settings. The examples provided in this chapter demonstrate some examples of environmental approaches often used with people with dementia. The Resources section provides additional information and resources used to help modify and enhance physical environments.

Conclusion

The Sensory Modulation Program (SMP) is a framework created to help families, caregivers, and professionals provide more nurturing and healing interventions to people experiencing mental health and cognitive challenges (Champagne 2011). This book provides adaptations to the SMP, to focus more specifically on its application with people with dementia. International initiatives related to providing care to people with dementia require an expansion of non-pharmacological options, including sensory-based approaches. The restraint reduction initiative also requires a more holistic approach to care delivery, and promotes sensory-based approaches for prevention and de-escalation purposes. The SMP provides information for families, caregivers, and professionals wanting to increase knowledge of sensory-based approaches for use at home or in health and nursing care settings. For more information on the SMP, see the Resources section.

Appendix A

Trauma Informed Safety Questionnaire

Name: _____ Date: _____

Traumatic experiences are those that have had an impact on a person over the course of their life. Please take a moment to identify whether any of the following apply and please provide as much information as possible (details, approximate year[s] or age[s] when the traumatic experience[s] occurred, and any other information that may be pertinent). Caregivers may assist the client or fully complete the Trauma Informed Safety Questionnaire when necessary.

Traumatic experiences:

☐ Physical abuse:

☐ Emotional abuse:

☐ Sexual abuse:

☐ Domestic abuse:

☐ War:

☐ Parent or loved one with mental illness:

☐ Significant losses:

☐ Medical trauma:

☐ Other(s):

Triggers:

- ☐ Loud noises:

- ☐ Touch:

- ☐ Scents:

- ☐ Sudden movements:

- ☐ Certain times of day:

- ☐ Certain songs or other things that may trigger memories, fears, or worries:

- ☐ Activities that may be triggering:

- ☐ Medical procedures that may be triggering:

- ☐ Other(s):

Warning signs: What does it look like when triggered?

- ☐ Sudden change(s) in behavior:

- ☐ Sudden change(s) in mood:

- ☐ Other(s):

Helpful strategy recommendations:

- ☐ Reassurance:

- ☐ Soothing techniques:

- ☐ Any particular sayings:

- ☐ Pictures or memory books:

- ☐ Religious or spiritual supports:

- ☐ Things to be sure NOT to do or say:

- ☐ Other(s):

Appendix B

Sensory Processing Caregiver Checklist

Adults and Older Persons

The Sensory Processing Caregiver Checklist was created to assist in identifying sensory processing patterns in adults or older persons with cognitive or communication difficulties. This is not a diagnostic tool and should be interpreted by a licensed professional with expertise in the area of sensory processing, in conjunction with clinical observations and further assessment as warranted.

This checklist helps to identify whether a person is displaying patterns that may be related to sensory modulation, discrimination, and/or motor performance. It is to be used for the purpose of information gathering to assist in the assessment process. This checklist is not meant to take the place of a formal assessment, but rather provides important information from the perspective of those who know the individual well to help inform the assessment process.

Sensory systems	High neurological threshold: (under-responsive or hypo-sensitive)	Low neurological threshold: (over-responsive or hyper-sensitive)	Sensory discrimination	Self-stimulatory or self-injurious behaviors
Movement (proprioception and vestibular)	☐ Prefers to be busy ☐ Prefers to be moving/being active ☐ Walks/paces a lot ☐ Tends to rock self ☐ Tends to chew on things ☐ Clenches things ☐ Bumps into things/clumsy ☐ Fidgets a lot ☐ Does not get dizzy easily ☐ Likes to dance or sway ☐ Tends to invade others' space ☐ Tends to use too much force with movements	☐ Tenses body when moved ☐ Becomes fearful or upset when moved ☐ Prefers being sedentary ☐ Does not like to be transferred ☐ Holds on really tight to people or to railings when walking or during transfers ☐ Gets dizzy or nauseous easily when moving or during car rides ☐ Fatigues easily ☐ Isolates ☐ Dislikes movement or exercise groups	☐ Clumsy/bumps into things a lot ☐ Requires postural support when seated ☐ Requires postural support during transfers ☐ Hesitates when going down stairs or through doorways ☐ Gets dizzy or nauseous easily when moving or during car rides ☐ Difficulty knowing how much force to use during movements ☐ Difficulty coordinating movements ☐ Difficulty getting in and out of chairs, the bed, or shower	☐ Head banging ☐ Hitting self ☐ Punching self ☐ Punching objects ☐ Forcefully grabs self or others ☐ Wringing skin ☐ Digging nails into self/others ☐ Throwing self out of chair or bed ☐ Isolating
Tactile	☐ Craves touch ☐ Likes hugs ☐ Is not bothered by being in close proximity to others ☐ Tends to pick up or touch things ☐ Does not mind getting hands messy during activities ☐ Does not mind grooming tasks ☐ Clingy behaviors ☐ Sometimes does not notice when touched ☐ Is not picky about the feeling of their clothing ☐ Higher pain tolerance	☐ Is bothered easily by being touched ☐ Rubs skin after touched ☐ Resists grooming (hair, shaving, tooth brushing, nail trimming) ☐ Does not like bathing or showering ☐ Does not like getting dressed/undressed ☐ Is bothered by getting hands, face, or other parts of the body messy ☐ Seems calmer when seated away from the proximity of others ☐ Bothered by tags or seams in clothing or by certain fabrics	☐ Finds it difficult or is slow to recognize the temperature of bath/shower water ☐ Seems to have a high pain tolerance ☐ Does not notice when touched unless can see or hear the person touching them ☐ Finds it difficult or is slow to recognize textures of fabric, food, art/craft supplies, or tactile qualities of other items	☐ Rubs or hits self after being touched ☐ Pinches self ☐ Scratches self ☐ Rubs skin to degree of harming self ☐ Picks at skin or other parts of the body

Auditory	☐ Does not seem bothered by noises ☐ Prefers the TV or radio to be turned up/kept on ☐ Does not mind making noise (use of instruments, singing, talking) ☐ May need instructions repeated ☐ Seeks out conversation ☐ Does not seem bothered by chaotic environments ☐ Makes different noises	☐ Dislikes noises ☐ Covers ears at times ☐ Dislikes activities involving a lot of noise (use of instruments, singing, talking) ☐ Asks for the volume of the TV, radio, or people's voices to lower ☐ Dislikes hearing the sounds of other people eating ☐ Avoids people who are loud and boisterous	☐ Demonstrates difficulty changing the volume of their voice to meet the appropriateness of the situation ☐ Asks for or needs to have information repeated ☐ Does not appear bothered by noisy environments ☐ Difficulty hearing when there are competing sounds in the environment ☐ Difficulty identifying where sounds are coming from	☐ Hits ears ☐ Screams when spoken to ☐ Becomes upset when the environment is noisy
Olfactory	☐ Seeks out scents or scented items ☐ Tends to smell things a lot ☐ Likes strong scents ☐ Does not notice mild scents	☐ Seems to be bothered by many scents ☐ Becomes irritable when exposed to certain scents ☐ Avoids strong scents ☐ Does not like items that are scented (soaps, lotions) ☐ Avoids certain foods due to the smell	☐ Tends to not notice scents ☐ Is not bothered by scents ☐ Has difficulty distinguishing between different scents	☐ Harms self when bothered by scent(s) ☐ Yells/screams when bothered by scent(s) ☐ Refuses to eat
Gustatory	☐ Seeks out food and drink ☐ Tends to taste things a lot ☐ Prefers foods with seasoning ☐ Mouths items a lot ☐ Does not notice changes in temperatures of food or drink unless extreme	☐ Seems to be bothered by any aspect of different types of oral stimuli (food texture, temperature, or type) ☐ Becomes irritable when exposed to certain foods ☐ Avoids food with seasonings ☐ Avoids certain types of food ☐ Picky eater	☐ Tends to not notice or enjoy the tastes of different types of food or drink ☐ Does not notice differences in food textures ☐ Does not notice differences in food temperature ☐ Has difficulty distinguishing between different foods	☐ Harms self when bothered by the tastes or textures of food ☐ Yells/screams when bothered by the tastes or textures of food ☐ Refuses to eat

(continued)

Sensory systems	High neurological threshold: (under-responsive or hypo-sensitive)	Low neurological threshold: (over-responsive or hyper-sensitive)	Sensory discrimination	Self-stimulatory or self-injurious behaviors
Vision	☐ Does not mind being in visually busy environments ☐ Likes to have the lights on ☐ Seeks out things to look at or watch ☐ Likes to be around a lot of people or activity ☐ Likes to watch TV or movies ☐ Likes to do tasks that require vision (puzzles, reading, mazes)	☐ Does not like to be in busy or chaotic environments ☐ Becomes irritable when exposed to bright lights ☐ Prefers low lighting ☐ Does not like sudden changes in lighting ☐ Rubs eyes often ☐ Squints a lot ☐ Gets watery eyes ☐ Prefers to wear sunglasses even indoors ☐ Avoids tasks involving visual searching (mazes, puzzles)	☐ May feel dizzy or sick when watching TV or movies with fast-paced or moving visual stimuli ☐ Tends to miss visual signs or details ☐ Difficulty with depth perception ☐ Appears to have difficulty with vision even with corrective lenses ☐ Difficulty finding clothing in drawers or closets (visually)	☐ Harms self when bothered by visual stimulation ☐ Yells/screams when bothered by visual stimulation

Bibliography

Allen, C.K., Earhart, C., & Blue, T. (1999). *Occupational therapy treatment goals for the physically and cognitively disabled.* Bethesda, MD: American Association of Occupational Therapy.

Alzheimer's Association (2017a). *What is dementia?* Accessed on 07/14/2017 at www.alz.org/what-is-dementia.asp.

Alzheimer's Association (2017b). *Hallucinations, delusions, and paranoia.* Accessed on 08/01/2015 at www.alz.org/national/documents/topicsheet_hallucinations.pdf.

Aman, E. & Thomas, D. (2008). Supervised exercise to reduce agitation in severely cognitively impaired persons. *Journal of the American Medical Directors Association, 10,* 271–276.

American Occupational Therapy Association (2008). *Frequently asked questions about Ayres sensory integration.* Accessed on 08/22/2017 at www.aota.org/~/media/Corporate/Files/Secure/Practice/Children/FAQAyres.pdf.

American Occupational Therapy Association (2011). *Occupational therapy using a sensory integration-based approach with adult populations.* Accessed on 08/22/2017 at www.aota.org/media/Corporate/Files/AboutOT/Professionals/WhatIsOT/CY/Fact-Sheets/FactSheet_SensoryIntegration.pdf.

American Occupational Therapy Association (2014). Occupational therapy practice framework: Domain and process, 3rd edition. *American Journal of Occupational Therapy, 68* (suppl. 1). Accessed on 08/22/2017 at http://ajot.aota.org/index.aspx.

Arnett, J. (1994). Sensation seeking: A new conceptualization and a new scale. *Personality and Individual Differences, 16*(2), 289–296. doi: 10.1016/0191-8869(94)90165-1.

Ayres, A.J. (1972). *Sensory integration and learning disorders.* Los Angeles, CA: Western Psychological Services.

Ayres, A.J. (1979). *Sensory integration and the child.* Los Angeles, CA: Western Psychological Services.

Ayres, A.J. (1989). *Sensory integration and praxis tests.* Los Angeles, CA: Western Psychological Services.

Ayres, A. J. (2005). *Sensory integration and the child: Understanding hidden sensory challenges*, revised edition. Los Angeles, CA: Western Psychological Services.

Azermai, M., Petrovic, M., Elseviers, M.M., Bourgeois, J., Van Bortel, L.M., & Vander Stichele, R.H. (2012). Systematic appraisal of dementia guidelines for the management of behavioural and psychological symptoms. *Ageing Research Reviews*, *11*(1), 78–86.

Baillon, S., Van Diepen, E., & Prettyman, R. (2002). Multi-sensory therapy in psychiatric care. *Advances in Psychiatric Treatment*, *8*(6), 444–450.

Baker, R., Bell, S., Baker, E., Holloway, J., Pearce, R., Dowling, Z., & Wareing, L.A. (2010). A randomized controlled trial of the effects of multi-sensory stimulation (MSS) for people with dementia. *British Journal of Clinical Psychology*, *40*(1), 81–96.

Baker, R., Holloway, J., Holtkamp, C., Larsson, A. *et al.* (2003). Effects of multi-sensory stimulation for people with dementia. *Journal of Advanced Nursing*, *43*(5), 465–477.

Ballard, C.G., O Brien, J.T., Reichelt, K., & Perry, E.K. (2002). Aromatherapy as a safe and effective treatment for the management of agitation in severe dementia: The results of a double-blind, placebo-controlled trial with Melissa. *Journal of Clinical Psychiatry*, *63*(7), 553–558.

Bera, D.R. (2008). Multisensory room and specialized dementia programming. *Nursing Homes Magazine*, *57*(2), 18.

Bidwell, J. (2009). *Agitation decision-making framework*. Accessed on 01/15/2018 at www.uws.edu. au/__data/assets/pdf_file/0007/76237/Agitation_Guidelines.pdf.

Blackburn, R. & Bradshaw, T. (2014). Music therapy for service users with dementia: A critical review of the literature. *Journal of Psychiatric and Mental Health Nursing*, *21*(10), 879–888.

Brown, C. & Dunn, W. (2002). *Adolescent/Adult Sensory Profile*. San Antonio, Texas: Pearson Assessment.

Brush, J.A. & Calkins, M.P. (2008). Cognitive impairment, wayfinding, and the long-term care environment. *Perspectives on Gerontology*, *13*, 65–73.

Burns, T. (2006). *Cognitive Performance Test*. Pequannock, NJ: Maddak.

Burns, A., Perry, E., Holmes, C., Francis, P. *et al.* (2011). A double-blind placebo-controlled randomized trial of Melissa officinalis oil and donepezil for the treatment of agitation in Alzheimer's disease. *Dementia and Geriatric Cognitive Disorders*, *31*(2), 158–164.

Cacchione, P. (2017). Sensory changes. Accessed on 07/14/2017 at https://consultgeri.org/geriatric-topics/sensory-changes.

Calkins, M. (2005). Building ideas: Environments for late-stage dementia. *Alzheimer's Care Quarterly*, *6*, 71–75.

Calkins, M., Szmerekovsky, J.G., & Biddle, S. (2007). Effect of increased time spent outdoors on individuals with dementia residing in nursing homes. *Journal of Housing for the Elderly*, *21*, 211–228.

Campellone, J. (2016). *Muscle atrophy*. NIH US National Library of Medicine, at https://medlineplus.gov/ency/article/003188.htm.

Canadian Foundation for Healthcare Improvement (CFHI) (2014). *CFHI supports projects to improve care for dementia patients: Teams across Canada will tackle inappropriate antipsychotic medication use.* Accessed on 08/01/2017 at www.cfhi-fcass.ca/SearchResultsNews/2014/06/04/cfhi-supports-projects-to-improve-care-for-dementia-patients-teams-across-canada-will-tackle-inappropriate-antipsychotic-medication-use.

Caspari, S., Eriksson, K., & Nåden, D. (2011). The importance of aesthetic surroundings: A study interviewing experts within different aesthetic fields. *Scandinavian Journal of Caring Sciences*, *25*, 134–142.

Ceccato, E., Vigato, G., Bonetto, C., Bevilacqua, A. *et al.* (2012). STAM protocol in dementia: A multicenter, single-blind, randomized, and controlled trial. *American Journal of Alzheimer's Disease and other Dementias*, *27*(5), 301–310.

Champagne, T. (2006). Creating sensory rooms: Environmental enhancements for acute inpatient mental health settings. *Mental Health Special Interest Section Quarterly*, *29*(4), 1–4.

Champagne, T. (2010). *Weighted blanket competency-based training program©*. Doctoral manuscript, Ann Arbor, Michigan.

Champagne, T. (2011). *Sensory modulation & environment: Essential elements of occupation.* Melbourne: Pearson Australia Group.

Champagne, T. (2017). *Sensory Modulation Program workbook: Adolescent and adult applications.* Florence, MA: Champagne Conferences & Consultation.

Champagne, T. & Stromberg, N. (2004). Sensory approaches in inpatient psychiatric settings: Innovative alternatives to seclusion and restraint. *Journal of Psychological Nursing*, *42*, 35–44.

Champagne, T., Mullen, B., Dickson, D., & Krishnamurty, S. (2015). Researching the safety and effectiveness of the weighted blanket with adults during an inpatient mental health hospitalization. *Occupational Therapy in Mental Health*, *31*, 211–233.

Chang, S., Chen, C., Shen, S., & Chiou, J. (2011). The effectiveness of an exercise programme for elders with dementia in a Taiwanese day-care centre. *International Journal of Nursing Practice*, *17*(3), 213–220.

Chatterton, W., Baker, F., & Morgan, K. (2010). The singer or the singing: Who sings individually to persons with dementia and what are the effects? *American Journal of Alzheimer's Disease & Other Dementias*, *25*(8), 641–649.

Chen, H.Y., Yang, H., Chi, H.J., & Chen, H.M. (2013). Physiological effects of deep pressure on anxiety alleviation: The weighted blanket approach. *Journal of Medical and Biological Engineering*, *33*, 463–470.

Chillot, R. (2013). *The power of touch.* Accessed on 08/01/2017 at www.psychologytoday.com/articles/201303/the-power-touch.

Chung, J.C., Lai, C.K., Chung, P.M., & French, H.P. (2002). Snoezelen for dementia. *Cochrane Library*, *4*, CD003152.

Cohen-Mansfield, J., Libin, A., & Marx, M.S. (2007). Non-pharmacological treatment of agitation: A controlled trial of systematic individualized intervention. *Journals of Gerontology Series A: Biological Sciences and Medical Sciences*, *62*, 908–916.

Collier, L., McPhearson, K., Ellis-Hill, C., Staal, J., & Bucks, R. (2010). Multisensory stimulation to improve functional performance in moderate to severe dementia: Interim results. *American Journal of Alzheimer's Disease & Other Dementias*, *25*(8), 698–703.

Connell, B.R., Sanford, J.A., & Lewis, D. (2007). Therapeutic effects of an outdoor activity program on nursing home residents with dementia. *Journal of Housing for the Elderly*, *21*, 195–209.

Cooke, M.L., Moyle, W., Shum, D.H., Harrison, S.D., & Murfield, J.E. (2010). A randomized controlled trial exploring the effect of music on agitated behaviours and anxiety in older people with dementia. *Aging and Mental Health*, *14*(8), 905–916.

Cowl, A.L. & Gaugler, J.E. (2014). Efficacy of creative arts therapy in treatment of Alzheimer's disease and dementia: A systematic literature review. *Activities, Adaptation & Aging, 38*(4), 281–330.

Cox, H., Burns, I., & Savage, S. (2004). Multi-sensory environments for leisure: Promoting well-being in nursing home residents with dementia. *Journal of Gerontological Nursing, 30*, 37–45.

Detweiler, M.B. & Warf, C. (2005). Dementia wander garden aids post cerebrovascular stroke restorative therapy: A case study. *Alternative Therapies in Health and Medicine, 11*, 54–58.

Doble, S. & Vania, C. (2009). Dementia. In B. Bonder & V.D. Bello-Hass (eds.) *Functional Performance in Older Adults* (pp. 216–227). Philadelphia, PA: F.A. Davis Co.

Doody, R.S., Stevens, J.C., Beck, C., Dubinsky, R.M. *et al.* (2001). Practice parameter: Management of dementia (an evidence-based review). *Journal of the American Academy of Neurology, 56*, 1154–1166.

Dowling, G.A., Graf, C.L., Hubbard, E.M., & Luxenberg, J.S. (2007). Light treatment for neuropsychiatric behaviors in Alzheimer's disease. *Western Journal of Nursing Research, 29*(8), 961–975.

Dunn, W. (2001). The sensations of everyday life: Theoretical, conceptual and pragmatic considerations. *American Journal of Occupational Therapy, 55*(6), 608–620.

Edwards, N.E., Beck, A. M., & Lim, E. (2014). Influence of aquariums on resident behavior and staff satisfaction in dementia units. *Western Journal of Nursing Research, 36*, 1309–1322.

El-Khoury, F., Cassou, B., Charles, M., & Molina, P. (2013). The effect of fall prevention exercise programmes on fall induced injuries in community dwelling older adults: Systematic review and meta-analysis of randomized controlled trials. *British Medical Journal, 347*, 1–13.

Fan, J.T. & Chen, K.M. (2011). Using silver yoga exercises to promote physical and mental health of elders with dementia in long-term care facilities. *International Psychogeriatrics, 23*(8), 1222–1230.

Fenech, A. & Baker, M. (2008). Casual leisure and the sensory diet: A concept for improving quality of life in neuropalliative conditions. *Neurorehabilitation, 23*, 369–376.

Folstein, M.F., Folstein, S.E., & McHugh, P.R. (1975). "Mini-Mental State": A practical method for grading the cognitive state of patients for the clinician. *Journal of Psychiatric Research, 12*, 189–198.

Forbes, R. & Gresham, M.D. (2011). Easing agitation in residents with "sundowning" behaviour. *Nursing & Residential Care, 13*(7), 345–347.

Forrester, L.T., Maayan, N., Orrell, M., Spector, A.E., Buchan, L.D., & Soares-Weiser, K. (2014). Aromatherapy for dementia. *The Cochrane Library, 2*, CD003150.

Freeman, W. (2000). *Neurodynamics: An exploration of mesoscopic brain dynamics.* London: Springer-Verlag.

Fu, C.Y., Moyle, W., & Cooke, M. (2013). A randomised controlled trial of the use of aromatherapy and hand massage to reduce disruptive behaviour in people with dementia. *BMC Complementary and Alternative Medicine, 13*, 1.

Fung, J.K.K., Tsang, H.W., & Chung, R.C. (2012). A systematic review of the use of aromatherapy in treatment of behavioral problems in dementia. *Geriatrics & Gerontology International, 12*(3), 372–382.

Geller, S.M. & Porges, S.W. (2014). Therapeutic presence: Neurophysiological mechanisms mediating feeling safe in therapeutic relationships. *American Psychological Association, 24*(3), 178–192.

Gigliotti, C.M. & Jarrott, S.E. (2005). Effects of horticultural therapy on engagement and affect. *Canadian Journal on Aging/La Revue Canadienne Du Vieillissement, 24*, 367–377.

Gitlin, L.N., Kales, H.C., & Lyketsos, C.G. (2012). Nonpharmacologic management of behavioral symptoms in dementia. Accessed on 08/01/2017 at http://jamanetwork.com/journals/jama/article-abstract/1392543.

Gonzalez, M.T. & Kirkevold, M. (2014). Benefits of sensory garden and horticultural activities in dementia care: A modified scoping review. *Journal of Clinical Nursing, 23*(19–20), 2698–2715.

Grant, C.F. & Wineman, J.D. (2007). The Garden-Use-Model: An environmental tool for increasing the use of outdoor space by residents with dementia in long-term care facilities. *Journal of Housing for the Elderly, 21*, 89–115.

Grasel, E., Wiltfang, J., & Kornhuber, J. (2003). Non-drug therapies for dementia: An overview of the current situation with regard to proof of effectiveness. *Dementia and Geriatric Cognitive Disorders, 15*, 115–125.

Haigh, J. & Mytton, C. (2016). Sensory interventions to support the wellbeing of people with dementia: A critical review. *British Journal of Occupational Therapy, 79*, 120–126.

Hammar, L.M., Emami, A., Engstrom, G., & Gotell, E. (2010). Reactions of persons with dementia to caregivers singing in morning care situations. *Open Nursing Journal, 4*, 35–41.

Hammar, L.M., Emami, A., Gotell, E., & Engstrom, G. (2011). The impact of caregivers' singing on expressions of emotion and resistance during morning care situations in persons with dementia: An intervention in dementia care. *Journal of Clinical Nursing, 20*, 969–978.

Hensman, M., Mudford, O.C., Dorrestein, M., & Brand, D. (2015). Behavioral evaluation of sensory-based activities in dementia care. *European Journal of Behavioral Analysis, 16*(2), 295–311.

Hernandez, R.O. (2007). Effects of therapeutic gardens in special care units for people with dementia: Two case studies. *Journal of Housing for the Elderly, 21*, 117–152.

Holmes, C., Hopkins, V., Hensford, C., MacLaughlin, V., Wilkinson, D., & Rosenvinge, H. (2002). Lavender oil as a treatment for agitated behaviour in severe dementia: A placebo controlled study. *International Journal of Geriatric Psychiatry, 17*(4), 305–308.

Hope, K.W. (1997). Using multi-sensory environments (MSEs) with people with dementia: Factors impeding their use as perceived by clinical staff. *Journal of Advanced Nursing, 25*, 780–785.

Hope, K.W. & Waterman, H.A. (1998). The effects of multisensory environments on older people with dementia. *Journal of Psychiatric and Mental Health Nursing, 5*, 377–385.

Hulme, C., Wright, J., Crocker, T., Oluboyede, Y., & House, A. (2010). Non-pharmacological approaches for dementia that informal carers might try or access: A systematic review. *International Journal of Geriatric Psychiatry, 25*, 756–763.

Hulsegge, J. & Verheul, A. (1986). *Snoezelen another world: A practical book of sensory experience environments for the mentally handicapped.* Chesterfield, UK: Rompa.

Janata, P. (2012). Effects of widespread and frequent personalized music programming on agitation and depression in assisted living facility residents with Alzheimer-type dementia. *Music and Medicine, 4*(1), 8–15.

Jarrott, S.E. & Gigliotti, C.M. (2010). Comparing responses to horticultural-based and traditional activities in dementia care programs. *American Journal of Alzheimer's Disease & Other Dementias, 25*, 657–665.

Jimbo, D., Kimura, Y., Taniguchi, M., Inoue, M., & Urakami, K. (2009). Effect of aromatherapy on patients with Alzheimer's disease. *Psychogeriatrics, 9*(4), 173–179.

Jootun, D. & McGhee, G. (2011). Effective communication with people who have dementia. *Nursing Standard, 25,* 40–46.

Katz, N., Averbuch, S., & Bar-Haim Erez, A. (2011). *Dynamic Lowenstein Occupational Therapy Cognitive Assessment Geriatric (DLOTCA–G)*. Pequannock, NJ: Maddak.

King, C. (2012). Managing agitated behavior in older people. *Nursing Older People, 24,* 33–36.

Klages, K., Zecevic, A., Orange, J.B., & Hobson, S. (2011). Potential of Snoezelen room multisensory stimulation to improve balance in individuals with dementia: A feasibility randomized controlled trial. *Clinical Rehabilitation, 25,* 607–616.

Kong, E.H., Evans, L.K., & Guevara, J.P. (2009). Nonpharmacological intervention for agitation in dementia: A systematic review and meta-analysis. *Aging & Mental Health, 13*(4), 512–520.

Kverno, K.S., Black, B.S., Nolan, M.T., & Rabins, P.V. (2009). Research on treating neuropsychiatric symptoms of advanced dementia with non-pharmacological strategies, 1998–2008: A systematic literature review. *International Psychogeriatrics, 21*(05), 825–843.

Lane, S.J., Smith Roley, S., & Champagne, T. (2014). Sensory integration and processing: Theory and applications to occupational performance. In B.B. Schell, G. Gillen, & M.J. Scaffa (eds.) *Willard and Spackman's Occupational Therapy*, 12th edition (pp. 816–868). Philadelphia, PA: Lippincott Williams & Wilkins.

Laver, K., Cumming, R., Dyer, S., Agar, M., Anstey, K., Beattie, E. *et al.* (2016). Clinical practice guidelines for dementia in Australia. *Medical Journal of Australia, 204,* 191–193.

LeBel, J. & Champagne, T. (2010). Integrating sensory and trauma-informed interventions: A Massachusetts state initiative, part 2. *Mental Health Special Interest Section Quarterly, 33*(2), 1–4.

Lee, H.S., Park, S.W., & Park, Y.J. (2016). Effects of physical activity programs on the improvement of dementia symptoms: A meta-analysis. *BioMed Research International,* 1–7. Accessed on 08/22/2017 at http://dx.doi.org/10.1155/2016/2920146.

Lee, Y. & Kim, S. (2008). Effects of indoor gardening on sleep, agitation, and cognition in dementia patients: A pilot study. *International Journal of Geriatric Psychiatry, 23,* 485–489.

Letts, L., Edwards, M., Berenyi, J., Moros, K. *et al.* (2011). Using occupations to improve quality of life, health and wellness, and client and caregiver satisfaction for people with Alzheimer's disease and related dementias. *American Journal of Occupational Therapy, 65*(5), 497–504.

Levin, M. (2016). *Weakness*. Accessed on 08/01/2017 at www.merckmanuals.com/professional/neurologic-disorders/symptoms-of-neurologic-disorders/weakness.

Lin, P.W.K., Chan, W.C., Ng, B.F.L., & Lam, L.C.W. (2007). Efficacy of aromatherapy (Lavandula angustifolia) as an intervention for agitated behaviours in Chinese older persons with dementia: A cross-over randomized trial. *International Journal of Geriatric Psychiatry, 22*(5), 405–410.

Lin, Y., Chu, H., Yang, C.Y., Chen, C.H. *et al.* (2011). Effectiveness of group music intervention against agitated behavior in elderly persons with dementia. *International Journal of Geriatric Psychiatry, 26*(7), 670–678.

Livingston, G., Kelly, L., Lewis-Holmes, E., Baio, G. *et al.* (2014). Non-pharmacological interventions for agitation in dementia: Systematic review of randomized controlled trials. *British Journal of Psychiatry, 205*(6), 436–442.

Locke, J.M. & Mudford, O.C. (2010). Using music to decrease disruptive vocalizations in a man with dementia. *Behavioral Interventions, 25*, 25–260.

MacLaughlin, J. & Stromberg, N. (2012). *Safety tools.* In J. LeBel & A. Lim (eds.) *Creating positive cultures of care: A resource guide,* 3rd edition. Boston, MA: Massachusetts Department of Mental Health.

Mahler, K. (2017). Interoception: The eighth sensory system. Lenexa, Kansas: AAPC Publishing.

Marquardt, G. (2011). Wayfinding for people with dementia: The role of architectural design. *Health Environments Research & Design Journal, 4*, 22–41.

Martin, L. (2016). *Aging changes in the senses.* Accessed on 06/20/2017 at https://medlineplus.gov/ency/article/004013.htm.

Maseda, A., Sánchez, A., Marante, M.P., González-Abraldes, I., Buján, A., & Millán-Calenti, J.C. (2014a). Effects of multisensory stimulation on a sample of institutionalized elderly people with dementia diagnosis: A controlled longitudinal trial. *American Journal of Alzheimer's Disease & Other Dementias, 29*, 463–473.

Maseda, A., Sánchez, A., Marante, M.P., González-Abraldes, I., de Labra, C., & Millán-Calenti, J.C. (2014b). Multisensory stimulation on mood, behavior, and biomedical parameters in people with dementia: Is it more effective than conventional one-to-one stimulation? *American Journal of Alzheimer's Disease & Other Dementias, 29*(7), 637–647.

May-Benson, T. (2014). *Adult/adolescent sensory history.* Newton, MA: Spiral Foundation.

McEvoy, P. & Plant, R. (2014). Dementia care: Using empathic curiosity to establish the common ground that is necessary for meaningful communication. *Journal of Psychiatric and Mental Health Nursing, 21*, 477–482.

Milev, R., Kellar, T., McLean, M., Mileva, V., Thompson, S., & Peever, L. (2008). Multisensory stimulation for elderly with dementia: A 24-week single-blind randomized controlled pilot study. *American Journal of Alzheimer's Disease & Other Dementias, 23*(4), 372–376.

Miller, L., Reisman, J., McIntosh, D., & Simon, J. (2001). An ecological model of sensory modulation. In S. Smith Roley, E. Blanche, & R. Schaaf (eds.) *Understanding the nature of sensory integration with diverse populations.* San Antonio, TX: Therapy Skill Builders.

Mullen, B., Champagne, T., Krishnamurty, S., Dickson, D., & Gao, R. (2008). Exploring the safety and therapeutic effects of deep pressure stimulation using a weighted blanket. *Occupational Therapy in Mental Health, 24*, 65–89.

Murphy, P.F., Miyazaki, Y., Detweiler, M.B., & Kim, K.Y. (2010). Longitudinal analysis of differential effects on agitation of a therapeutic wander garden for dementia patients based on ambulation ability. *Dementia, 9*, 355–373.

National Association of State Mental Health Program Directors (NASMHPD) (2000). NASMHPD position statement on services and supports to trauma survivors. Accessed on 08/22/2017 at www.nasmhpd.org/sites/default/files/I_1_A_NASMHPD_TraumaPosition Statement.pdf.

National Coalition of Auditory Processing Disorders (2017). *What is auditory processing disorder?* Accessed on 08/01/2017 at www.ncapd.org/What_is_APD_.html.

National Executive Training Institute (2003, 2009). *Creating violence free and coercion free treatment environments for the reduction of seclusion and restraint.* Workshop presentations. Boston, MA/Alexandria, VA: National Technical Assistance Center for State Mental Health Planning.

National Institute for Health and Care Excellence (NICE) (2017). *Dementia resources.* Accessed on 08/01/2017 at www.nice.org.uk/search?q=dementia.

Oken, B.S., Zajdel, D., Kishiyama, S., Flegal, K. *et al.* (2006). Randomized, controlled, six-month trial of yoga in healthy seniors: Effects on cognition and quality of life. *Alternative Therapies in Health and Medicine, 12,* 40.

Padilla, R. (2011). Effectiveness of environment-based interventions for people with Alzheimer's disease and related dementias. *American Journal of Occupational Therapy, 65,* 514–522.

Parham, L.D., Smith Roley, S., May-Benson, T., Koomar, J., Brett-Green, B., Burke, J.P., Cohn, E.S., Mailloux, Z., Miller, L.J., & Schaaf, R.C. (2011). Development of a fidelity measure for research on effectiveness of Ayres Sensory Integration® intervention. *American Journal of Occupational Therapy, 65,* 2, 133–142.

Perkins, J., Bartlett, H., Travers, C., & Rand, J. (2008). Dog-assisted therapy for older people with dementia: A review. *Australian Journal on Ageing, 27,* 177–182.

Pitkälä, K., Savikko, N., Poysti, M., Strandberg, T., & Laakkonen, M. (2013). Efficacy of physical exercise intervention on mobility and physical functioning in older people with dementia: A systematic review. *Experimental Gerontology, 48,* 85–93.

Pöllänen, S.H. & Hirsimäki, R.M. (2014). Crafts as memory triggers in reminiscence: A case study of older women with dementia. *Occupational Therapy in Health Care, 28*(4), 410–430.

Press-Sandler, O., Freud, T., Volkov, I., Peleg, R., & Press, Y. (2016). Aromatherapy for the treatment of patients with behavioral and psychological symptoms of dementia: A descriptive analysis of RCTs. *Journal of Alternative and Complementary Medicine, 22,* 422–428.

Reimer, M.A., Slaughter, S., Donaldson, C., Currie, G., & Eliasziw, M. (2004). Special care facility compared with traditional environments for dementia care: A longitudinal study of quality of life. *Journal of the American Geriatrics Society, 52,* 1085–1092.

Reisman, J.E. & Hanschu, B. (1992). *Sensory integration inventory–revised for individuals with developmental disabilities: User's guide.* Hugo, MN: PDP Press.

Responsible Reform for the Middle Class (2010). *Patient protection and affordable care act: Detailed summary.* Accessed on 08/22/2017 at www.dpc.senate.gov/healthreformbill/healthbill04.pdf.

Riley-Doucet, C.K. (2009). Use of multisensory environments in the home for people with dementia. *Journal of Gerontological Nursing, 35*(5), 42–52.

Robinson, L., Hutchings, D., Dickinson, H.O., Corner, L. *et al.* (2007). Effectiveness and acceptability of non-pharmacological interventions to reduce wandering in dementia: A systematic review. *International Journal of Geriatric Psychiatry, 22*(1), 9–22.

Rolland, Y., Pillard, F., Klapouszczak, A., Reynish, E. *et al.* (2007). Exercise program for nursing home residents with Alzheimer's disease: A 1-year randomized, controlled trial. *Journal of the American Geriatrics Society, 55*(2), 158–165.

Rosen, W.G., Mohs, R.C., & Davis, K.L. (1984). A new rating scale for Alzheimer's disease. *American Journal of Psychiatry, 141,* 1356–1364.

Sánchez, A., Millan-Calenti, J.C., Lorenzo-Lopez, L., & Maseda, A. (2013). Multisensory stimulation for people with dementia: A review of the literature. *American Journal of Alzheimer's Disease & Other Dementias, 28,* 7–14.

Staal, J.A., Amanda, S., Matheis, R., Collier, L., Calia, T., Hanif, H., & Kofman, E. S. (2007). The effects of Snoezelen (multi-sensory behavior therapy) and psychiatric care on agitation, apathy, and activities of daily living in dementia patients on a short term geriatric psychiatric inpatient unit. *International Journal of Psychiatry in Medicine, 37*(4), 357–370.

Teeple, R.C., Caplan, J.P., & Stern, M.D. (2009). Visual hallucinations: Differential diagnosis and treatment. *Primary Care Companion to the Journal of Clinical Psychiatry, 11*, 26–32.

US Department of Health and Human Services (2013). *National plan to address Alzheimer's disease.* Accessed on 08/01/2017 at http://aspe.hhs.gov/daltcp/napa/natlplan.shtml#strategy1.B.

US Food and Drug Administration (2013). *Information for healthcare professionals: Conventional antipsychotics.* Accessed on 08/01/2017 at www.fda.gov/drugs/drugsafety/postmarketdrugsa fetyinformationforpatientsandproviders/ucm124830.html.

Vasionytė, I. & Madison, G. (2013). Musical intervention for patients with dementia: A meta-analysis. *Journal of Clinical Nursing, 22*(9–10), 1203–1216.

Venturelli, M., Scarsini, R., & Schena, F. (2011). Six-month walking program changes cognitive and ADL performance in patients with Alzheimer. *American Journal of Alzheimer's Disease & Other Dementias, 26*(5), 381–388.

Veselinova, C. (2014). Influencing communication and interaction in dementia. *Nursing & Residential Care, 16*, 162–166.

Vestibular Disorders Association (2017). *The human balance system: A complex coordination of central and peripheral systems.* Accessed on 08/01/2017 at http://vestibular.org/sites/default/files/page_files/Documents/Human%20Balance%20System.pdf.

Victoria State Government (2017). *Designing for people with dementia.* Accessed on 08/01/2017 at www2.health.vic.gov.au/ageing-and-aged-care/dementia-friendly-environments/desigining-for-dementia.

Vreugdenhil, A., Cannell, J., Davies, A., & Razay, G. (2012). A community-based exercise programme to improve functional ability in people with Alzheimer's disease: A randomized controlled trial. *Scandinavian Journal of Caring Sciences, 26*, 12–19.

Vries, K. de (2013). Communicating with older people with dementia. *Nursing Older People, 25*, 30–37.

Ward-Smith, P., Llanque, S.M., & Curran, D. (2009). The effect of multisensory stimulation on persons residing in an extended care facility. *American Journal of Alzheimer's Disease & Other Dementias, 24*(6), 450–455.

Weert, J.C. van, Kerkstra, A., van Dulmen, A.M., Bensing, J.M., Peter, J.G., & Ribbe, M. W. (2004). The implementation of Snoezelen in psychogeriatric care: An evaluation through the eyes of caregivers. *International Journal of Nursing Studies, 41*(4), 397–409.

Wilbarger, P. (1995). The sensory diet: Activity programs based upon sensory processing theory. *Sensory Integration Special Interest Section Quarterly, 18*(2), 1–4.

Williams, E. & Jenkins, R. (2008). Dog visitation therapy in dementia care: A literature review. *Nursing Older People, 20*(8), 31–35.

Wood, W., Womack, J., & Hooper, B. (2009). Dying of boredom: An exploratory case study of time use, apparent affect, and routine activity situations on two Alzheimer's special care units. *American Journal of Occupational Therapy, 63*, 337–350.

Yamaguchi, H., Maki, Y., & Yamagami, T. (2010). Overview of non-pharmacological interventions for dementia and principles of brain-activating rehabilitation. *Psychogeriatrics, 10*, 206–213.

Resources

Activity-related resources

- DementiaKT Hub: http://dementiakt.com.au/?ct=1
- Golden Carers: www.goldencarers.com
- Montessori Australia: http://montessorifordementia.com.au
- Senior fitness exercises: https://eldergym.com/elderly-balance.html

Alzheimer's and dementia organizations

- Alzheimer's Australia: www.fightdementia.org.au
- American Alzheimer's Association: www.alz.org
- Alzheimer's Association (2017). Interactive brain tour explaining how the brain works and the effects of Alzheimer's disease. Available in different languages: www.alz.org/alzheimers_disease_4719.asp
- Alzheimer's Association (2017). Ten warning signs of Alzheimer's disease: www.alz.org/national/documents/tenwarnsigns.pdf
- *Alzheimer's & Dementia®: The Journal of the Alzheimer's Association*, open access online journal
- Alzheimer's Foundation: www.alzfdn.org
- Centers for Disease Control: Alzheimer's Disease: www.cdc.gov/aging/aginginfo/alzheimers.htm
- National Health and Medical Research Council: Australian Clinical Practice Guidelines: https://clinicalguidelines.gov.au
- National Institute on Aging: www.nia.nih.gov/health/alzheimers
- National Institute for Health and Care Excellence: www.nice.org.uk/guidance/qs86

Canadian initiatives

- Canadian Foundation for Healthcare Improvement (CFHI): www.cfhi-fcass.ca/SearchResultsNews/2016/05/16/new-national-results-taking-seniors-off-antipsychotics-shows-dramatic-improvement-in-care

- Windsor Star care homes: http://windsorstar.com/news/local-news/kicking-the-antipsychotic-drug-habit-at-long-term-care-homes

Caregiver and family resources

- Community Organization Practice Tool: www.actonalz.org/sites/default/files/documents/ACT-Provider-CommunityPracticeTool.pdf

- Know the Signs: Early Detection Matters: www.alz.org/national/documents/tenwarnsigns.pdf

- Managing dementia across the continuum (mid to late stage): www.actonalz.org/sites/default/files/documents/ACT-Provider-ManagingDementia.pdf

- Stages of Alzheimer's: www.alz.org/alzheimers_disease_stages_of_alzheimers.asp

Evaluation- and assessment-related resources

- Common dementia-related assessment scales: www.assessmentpsychology.com/geriatricscales.htm

- Agitation Decision Making Framework: www.uws.edu.au/__data/assets/pdf_file/0007/76237/Agitation_Guidelines.pdf

- KAER Toolkit: 4-Step Process to Detecting Cognitive Impairment and Early Diagnosis of Dementia

- Teepa Snow's Positive Approach to Brain Change: http://teepasnow.com/about/about-teepa-snow

Physical environments

- American Association of Multisensory Environments: www.aamse.us

- Creating Multisensory Environments for People with Dementia: Guide Book http://fada.kingston.ac.uk/de/MSE_design_in_dementia_care/doc/How%20to%20make%20a%20Sensory%20Room%20for%20people%20with%20dementia.pdf

- Designing for people with dementia: www2.health.vic.gov.au/ageing-and-aged-care/dementia-friendly-environments/strategies-checklists-tools/home-like-environment

- Dementia and enabling environments:
  - www.enablingenvironments.com.au
  - www.enablingenvironments.com.au/uploads/5/0/4/5/50459523/harmfulplants.pdf
  - International Snoezelen Association: https://snoezelen-professional.com/en

- Sensory gardens:
  - Sensory Trust: www.sensorytrust.org.uk/information/factsheets/sensory-garden-1.html
  - Enabling gardens: www.fightdementia.org.au/sites/default/files/1.-Alz-Aust-Conference-2013.pdf
  - Gardens that Care: Planning Outdoor Environments for People with Dementia: http://dbmas.org.au/uploads/resources/101796_ALZA_Garden32pp_LR.pdf

Restraint reduction

- NASMHPD's six core strategies: www.nasmhpd.org/sites/default/files/Consolidated%20 Six%20Core%20Strategies%20Document.pdf
- Massachusetts Department of Mental Health (2010). *Seclusion/restraint reduction initiative resources*: www.mass.gov/eohhs/gov/departments/dmh/restraintseclusion-reduc- tion-initiative.html
- Occupational therapy's role in restraint and seclusion reduction: www.aota.org/-/media/ Corporate/Files/AboutOT/Professionals/WhatIsOT/MH/Facts/Restraint%20fact%20sheet. pdf
- OT Innovations: www.ot-innovations.com
- SAMHSA's concept of trauma and guidance for a trauma informed care approach: http:// store.samhsa.gov/shin/content/SMA14-4884/SMA14-4884.pdf
- Te Pou's sensory modulation and restraint reduction resources: www.tepou.co.nz/library/ tepou/sensorymodulation

Sensory integration and processing

- Ayres Sensory Integration®: www.siglobalnetwork.org
- OT Innovations: www.ot-innovations.com
- Sensory processing:
  - Hearing and balance crash course: www.youtube.com/watch?v=Ie2j7GpC4JU
  - The nervous system: www.youtube.com/watch?v=x4PPZCLnVkA
  - Taste and smell: www.youtube.com/watch?v=mFm3yA1nslE
- Sensory processing disorder:
  - A child's view of sensory processing: www.youtube.com/watch?v=D1G5ssZlVUw
  - Star Institute: www.spdstar.org/basic/understanding-sensory-processing-disorder

Videos

- *Alive Inside* by Dan Cohen (2014), documentary on the use of music with people with dementia
- How Alzheimer's changes the brain: www.nia.nih.gov/health/video-how-alzheimers- changes-brain

Stages of dementia and Alzheimer's: www.khanacademy.org/science/health-and-medicine/ mental-health/dementia-delirium-alzheimers/v/stages-of-dementia-and-alzheimers-disease

Index